Casebook for *DSM-5*®

Elizabeth Ventura, PhD, LPL, NCC, is a counselor educator, qualitative researcher, and trauma specialist. She has been practicing clinically since 2004 and has specific clinical training in both cognitive behavioral therapy and dialectical behavioral therapy. Although her area of expertise focuses on trauma work and the treatment of eating disorders, she has built her clinical practice working with individuals across the life span where she has experience in various mental health conditions. She is a core faculty member in the clinical mental health counseling department at Walden University. Her teaching experience includes such courses as psychopathology and diagnosis, research design and program evaluation, testing and appraisal, advanced counseling techniques, foundations of counseling, counseling trauma survivors, practicum, internship, and supervision.

Dr. Ventura has presented at numerous local, state, and national conferences, including the profession's flagship professional conferences, the American Counseling Association and the Association for Counselor Education and Supervision. She has published chapters in such texts as *Trauma Counseling: Theories and Interventions; The Counselor's Companion: What Every Beginning Counselor Needs to Know;* and the forthcoming *Introduction to the Counseling Profession.* In addition, she is the president of Associates in Counseling & Wellness, LLC, which provides private therapy and group therapy services to individuals, families, and couples.

Casebook for *DSM-5*®
Diagnosis and Treatment Planning

Elizabeth Ventura, PhD, LPL, NCC

Editor

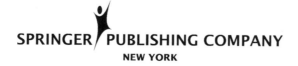

SPRINGER PUBLISHING COMPANY
NEW YORK

Springer Publishing Company, LLC
11 West 42nd Street
New York, NY 10036
www.springerpub.com

Acquisitions Editor: Nancy Hale
Compositor: S4Carlisle Publishing Services

ISBN: 978-0-8261-2752-5
e-book ISBN: 978-0-8261-2753-2

16 17 18 19 20/5 4 3 2 1

The author and the publisher of this Work have made every effort to use sources believed to be reliable to provide information that is accurate and compatible with the standards generally accepted at the time of publication. The author and publisher shall not be liable for any special, consequential, or exemplary damages resulting, in whole or in part, from the readers' use of, or reliance on, the information contained in this book. The publisher has no responsibility for the persistence or accuracy of URLs for external or third-party Internet websites referred to in this publication and does not guarantee that any content on such websites is, or will remain, accurate or appropriate.

Library of Congress Cataloging-in-Publication Data

Names: Ventura, Elizabeth, editor.
Title: Casebook for DSM-5® : diagnosis and treatment planning / editor,
    Elizabeth Ventura, PhD, LPL, NCC.
Description: New York : Springer Publishing Company, [2017] | Includes
    bibliographical references and index.
Identifiers: LCCN 2016041733 | ISBN 9780826127525
Subjects: LCSH: Diagnostic and statistical manual of mental disorders. 5th
    ed. | Anxiety disorders—Diagnosis. | Anxiety disorders—Treatment.
Classification: LCC RC531 .C36 2017 | DDC 616.85/220076—dc23
LC record available at https://lccn.loc.gov/2016041733

Printed in the United States of America by Gasch Printing.

Contents

Contributors   *vii*
Preface   *ix*
Acknowledgments   *xi*
Introduction   *xiii*

Dylan   *1*

Carol   *7*

Keith   *13*

Carla   *19*

Todd   *23*

John   *27*

Michael   *33*

Jamie   *39*

Maria   *43*

Jessica   *45*

Rhonda   *55*

Jeremy   *65*

Dan   *71*

Tim   *75*

Mike   *79*

George   *83*

Jonathan   *89*

Julia   *95*

Cate   *99*

Alec   *105*

Billy   *109*

Jack   *117*

Luz   *123*

Nathan   *131*

Bryant   *135*

Adrienne   *139*

Jacob   *143*

Jason   *149*

Bashir   *155*

Index   *159*

Contributors

Heather Ambrose, PhD, LCMHC, LMFT
Core Faculty, School of Counseling, Walden University, Layton, Utah

Renee Anderson, PhD, LPCC-S
Core Faculty, School of Counseling, Walden University, Butler, Pennsylvania

Brooks Bastian Hanks, PhD, LCPC
Core Faculty, School of Counseling, Walden University, Southeast Idaho

Jayna Bonfini, MA, LPC, NCC
Private Practice, McMurray, Pennsylvania

Christian J. Dean, PhD, LPC, LMFT, NCC
Core Faculty, School of Counseling, Walden University, Baton Rouge, Louisiana

Jeannie Falkner, PhD, LCSW
Core Faculty, Walden University, Oxford, Mississippi

Brandy L. Gilea, PhD, LPCC-S, NCC
Core Faculty, Walden University, Canfield, Ohio

Maranda A. Griffin, PhD, LPC
Core Faculty, Walden University, Orange Park, Florida

Christie Jenkins, PhD, LPCC-S
Core Faculty, School of Counseling, Walden University, Perrysburg, Ohio

Sola Kippers, PhD, LPC-S, LMFT
Clinical Counseling, Capella University, Baton Rouge, Louisiana

Rhonda Neswald-Potter, PhD, LPCC, ACS
Clinical Director, Manzanita Counseling Center, University of New Mexico, Contributing Faculty Member, Walden University, Albuquerque, New Mexico

Rachel M. O'Neill, PhD, LPCC-S
Core Faculty, MS in Clinical Mental Health Counseling Program, Walden University, Poland, Ohio

Stacy Overton, PhD, LPC, LAC
Core Faculty, Walden University, Fort Collins, Colorado

Joshua Parnell, BA
Student, Walden University, Pittsburgh, Pennsylvania

Torey Portrie-Bethke, PhD
NCC, Core Faculty, School of Counseling, Walden University, Northwood, New Hampshire

Amanda Rovnak, PhD, PCC-S, LICDC-CS, LISW-S
Core Faculty Member, School of Counseling, Walden University, Copley, Ohio

Jessica Russo, PhD, LPCC-S, NCC
Core Faculty, School of Counseling, Walden University, Portage Lakes, Ohio

Stephanie L. Stern, MA, LPC, LBS, NCC
Private Practice, McMurray, Pennsylvania

Elizabeth M. Ventura, PhD, LPC, NCC
Core Faculty, School of Counseling, Walden University, McMurray, Pennsylvania

Margaret Zappitello, EdD, LPC, LMFT, LAC, MAC, NCC
Core Faculty, School of Counseling, Walden University, Brighton, Colorado

Preface

The collection of cases presented in this book has been compiled from seasoned clinicians who have experienced complex client symptomology. These cases illustrate real-world examples of actual clients seen in practice. The details of the cases are organized to provide readers with examples of case conceptualization, as well as diagnostic impressions, conclusions, and treatment recommendations. Remembering that each client is different, and the training and skill level of the treating therapist is equally unique, the recommendations provided in the cases serve as examples for students to critically analyze and adapt their own theoretical approach when conceptualizing the cases.

It is certainly true for me that the clients I have encountered have changed my life. The gratefulness and gratitude I feel for having the opportunity to walk with each of them throughout their personal journeys is inexpressible. Through my own work with clients I have learned that authenticity cannot be attempted; rather, it must be interwoven into the fabric of the self. For 50 minutes, we are given the gift to sit across from another human being struggling deeply with aspects of his or her life and are entrusted to help him or her navigate this pain. We are entrusted to know the way, sometimes as a guide, other times as a follower. Regardless of the role we play, we are entrusted to be among the few that see this level of human vulnerability and shame in its most exposed state. We are expected to be prepared for this and to meet it with passion, integrity, and competence.

Practice now for those moments on the horizon.

■ RECOMMENDATIONS FOR USE

This casebook provides a practical and realistic way for students in such mental health professions as clinical psychology, counseling psychology, counseling, and social work to put the new *DSM-5* into practice by presenting actual clinical experiences from practitioners. By exploring detailed clinical vignettes, this text offers trainees the opportunity to explore their own ideas on symptom presentation, diagnosis, and treatment planning with a full range of disorders and conditions covered in the *DSM-5*. Unlike other casebooks, this book not only provides vignettes, but also explores the rationale behind diagnostic criteria and connects diagnostic criteria in the *DSM-5* with symptomology in the case. In addition, each case includes a discussion of treatment interventions that is crucial for students in helping professions. These treatment considerations are inclusive of a wide range of evidence-based approaches as appropriate for each case. Cases are presented across major categories of disorders to help students understand the nature of differential diagnosis. Cases also reflect cultural and social considerations in making diagnostic decisions.

An ideal text to enhance courses in psychopathology and diagnosis, as well as practicum and internship, this casebook will diversify and broaden the classroom experience by enlightening students with compelling clinical cases that have been experienced by practicing professionals.

Elizabeth M. Ventura

Acknowledgments

Thanks are due to the countless individuals who are brave enough to seek counseling and whose stories have inspired this book. These individuals may never fully understand how their stories can help change the lives of others and how their resilience has changed mine. I am grateful every day for having been a part of each of their journeys.

As clinicians, we advocate for self-care and a work–life balance. My husband, Mick, is my balance and truly the best human being I know. Thank you for giving me the time, encouragement, and love to make this happen.

Last, I am overwhelmed by the support of my colleagues and the contributions made by the incredibly talented clinicians who have provided the cases in this book.

Introduction

The *Diagnostic and Statistical Manual of Mental Disorders*, Fifth Edition (*DSM-5*; American Psychiatric Association. 2013) is the result of the first significant revision since the publication of *DSM-IV* in 1994. With advances in research and clinical applications, modifications were needed to accurately frame client symptom presentation and reflect the changes and advances in science and technology, as well as cultural and societal factors. With these changes come a set of standards that practitioners-in-training should familiarize themselves with and learn to accurately apply diagnostic criteria to real-world examples.

As a counselor educator, I have found that the use of diagnostic criteria in the absence of practical case applications is limiting for students. The power of using real-world case presentations to help students conceptualize symptomology helps trainees to integrate knowledge in a way that surpasses traditional rote memory learning strategies.

Counselor educators have an ethical responsibility to act as gatekeepers in training programs. Although professionalism and comportment issues are foundational elements in our profession, competence in the areas of diagnosis and theory-driven interventions have risen to the surface with managed care. Often, in short periods of time, change is expected. Counselors-in-training are charged with implementing theory and technique with intentionality to arrive at the correct diagnosis and treatment plan in order to effectively deliver care. This is certainly a task that requires confidence, competence, and creativity. Research has shown that trainees gain a sense of efficacy from practicing in supervisory settings with realistic examples and from a constructivist paradigm. The hope is that this book can begin the process for trainees to understand the client complexities that present daily in the counseling office and meet those challenges with a sense of self-assurance that can, in fact, help to promote change.

■ REFERENCES

American Psychiatric Association. (2013). *Diagnostic and statistical manual of mental disorders* (5th ed.). Arlington, VA: American Psychiatric Publishing.
American Psychiatric Association. (1994). *Diagnostic and statistical manual of mental disorders* (4th ed.). Washington, DC: Author.

Dylan

■ HISTORY

Dylan attended his first session accompanied by his 42-year-old mother, Brenda, and 22-year-old sister, Carly. As a 15-year-old freshman in Cyber High school, Dylan was incredibly attached to his family and relied on his sister and mom as his primary supports.

A week prior to his initial appointment, Brenda called for a phone consultation to discuss Dylan's primary symptoms. At the time of the call, Dylan was not eating a majority of foods that were prepared at home. He was struggling to leave the house and seemed affected by preoccupation with thoughts around getting the stomach flu. Dylan was fearful that eating anything that was prepared at home would result in vomiting and prolonged illness. He would routinely inspect utensils at home to ensure cleanliness and oversee his parents and siblings as they participated in preparing meals. With the severity of symptoms increasing over the course of 60 days, Dylan had lost 17 pounds as a result of the eating restrictions. Brenda had notified me that his current psychologist attributed the symptoms to anxiety; however, he was not seeing any alleviation of symptoms despite weekly therapy.

As Dylan entered the office, he slipped his sleeve over his hand to open the door from the lobby to the main office but then quickly recovered and extended his hand to accept the clipboard of paperwork and pencil to finish the logistics of the intake appointment. He made very little eye contact throughout the session, and his responses were literal. Questions such as, "Tell me what has been going on" required extensive further clarification because the lack of clarity in the initial question caused intense anxiety. Dylan often looked to his mother and sister throughout the session to assist in answering questions or for clarification; however, he did correct any misinterpretations that they expressed. He was able to discuss his interests in video gaming and design, online role-playing games, and Lego building but expressed that all of these are better when interacting with others online. Although Dylan wants peer interaction and friendships, his past experience has been such that he now avoids the inevitable rejection that comes with attempting social interactions.

At numerous points throughout the intake, Dylan coughed repeatedly as he listened to his mother and sister describe the tumultuous relationship he has with his older brother, Corey, who recently returned home from college. Corey, 19, is described as having little empathy and time for Dylan's anxiety and, as a result, takes a very harsh approach with Dylan that creates stress and arguments. Dylan sleeps on the bottom bunk, with Corey often climbing over him at odd times of the night, disrupting his routine, as he has no schedule since being home from school. As Dylan discussed a recent argument over "rocking the bed," his cough became more pronounced and repetitive. Brenda discussed that Dylan has always "rocked" himself to sleep, and although this would not be much of an issue in and of itself, it poses quite an issue being on the bottom of a bunk bed.

The intake progressed to discuss more of the symptoms related to his weight loss. Dylan discussed feeling that the weight loss now was likely unhealthier than any stomach flu he could ever contract. He had no rational reason for fearing vomiting, nor could he describe a situation in which someone died from profuse vomiting. When asked, "What is the worst thing that could happen to you?" he was speechless and yet, strangely enough, a sense of calmness overcame him realizing he did not know the worst case scenario.

Dylan coughed again. And again. And again.

Brenda commented that the coughing occurs daily and reported that it has been "happening forever." Carly reported that it has not always been coughing; he has had sniffling episodes during which he has sounded sick but was perfectly healthy.

More social history from Dylan's past reveals that he has struggled with appropriate communication that is relevant to his peer group. He has a difficult time dealing with rule breakers and has always been incredibly literal. When asked, "What would you say if I told you it was raining cats and dogs outside?" He responded, "I would first look outside to see what you were referring to and make sure there were not cats or dogs outside." Brenda and Carly both agreed that his inability to connect to other kids his age in socially appropriate activities has caused a tremendous amount of isolation in his life.

■ DIAGNOSTIC IMPRESSIONS

Dylan has accepted that his life, as it stands, is not worth living. He fears a life in which he is afraid to eat food prepared by another individual and wants to understand why he allows these "thoughts to take over my mind." His preoccupation with flu symptoms and vomiting creates a world in which he needs to compensate by attempting to create rules so that it does not happen. These rules are irrational and change according to the needs he may have at the time. For example, Dylan will not eat red meat prepared by his mother in his kitchen at home; however, if his sister agrees to make his dinner and it is red meat, he will eat it. He will eat out at certain restaurants with buffets, but not others. Having these rules in place gives Dylan a sense of control and this, in turn, creates a sense of safety for him that feels comfortable, but only for a moment.

Dylan is still in a place where he wants to appear somewhat socially acceptable. He secretly attempted to open the door with his sleeve; however, he quickly recovered to take the pencil and intake paperwork (although he was thinking of washing his hands the entire time the session was conducted).

His obsessions (thoughts of getting sick, contaminated, or infected) are consuming, and his quality of life has deteriorated. As a result of these obsessive thoughts, he engages in repetitive compulsive behaviors that include checking food temperatures, cleaning utensils, hand washing to the point of raw skin, and checking kitchen cleanliness. Despite his best efforts, he cannot control the urges he feels and rarely gets a break from the obsessive thoughts and compulsions that accompany them.

Motor tics co-occur often in individuals with Obsessive-Compulsive Disorder (OCD). These tics occur nearly every day and have occurred prior to the age of 18. Individuals experiencing these tics find that they are uncontrollable and involuntary. Co-occurrence of these two conditions has been fairly high with more than 60% of individuals with Tic Disorder experiencing symptoms of OCD.

Dylan has experienced distress related to social relationships prior to the manifestation of the OCD symptoms. He makes little eye contact, struggles to understand social cues and nonverbal body language, and has difficulty relating to his peer group despite wanting to have friendships. Dylan fixates easily on issues or behaviors and has a difficult time with inferences or interpreting meaning. Given the symptoms presentation, there should be more diagnostic testing to determine if an Autism Spectrum Disorder is warranted.

■ DIAGNOSTIC CONCLUSIONS

> Obsessive-Compulsive Disorder (OCD)
> Tic Disorder
> Social (Pragmatic) Communication Disorder

■ SUGGESTED THERAPEUTIC INTERVENTIONS

OCD and Tic Disorder are neuropsychiatric disorders that are often treated by behavior modification and/or medication management. In both cases, parental and/or familial support is also indicative of long-term success rates in those diagnosed. According to Lombroso and Scahill (2008), habit reversal training (HRT) "involves helping clients increase awareness of tics prior to their expression, self-monitoring, relaxation training, and competing responses." Individuals aware of an expression of a tic are encouraged to produce a voluntary competing response instead of the conditioned response. Early indications show that this is a positive behavior modification for those suffering from Tic Disorders.

The treatment of OCD has been well established in the roots of behavioral therapy. Exposing clients to the feared stimuli and blocking the conditioned response ultimately reduces the symptoms and severity of OCD. In children and adolescents, it is imperative that parent training is reinforced so that the child can have continued support at home and/or school. In either case, medication management coupled with behavior modification is generally considered the most comprehensive treatment protocol.

■ FOR YOUR CONSIDERATION

1. Given what you know about Dylan, what are some ways you can begin to help him understand his own diagnoses? Considering that certain concepts related to his condition may be confusing, be creative in your approach!
2. How might Dylan's family hinder his progress with his OCD in the home environment? Consider ways to help his family support him and not enable him.

■ REFERENCE

Lombroso, P. J., & Scahill, L. (2008). Tourette syndrome and obsessive-compulsive disorder. *Brain Development, 4*, 231–237.

Carol

■ HISTORY

Carol is a 36-year-old Caucasian female who is presenting to outpatient counseling after being referred by her probation officer. Carol is a legally involved client with an extensive criminal history involving solicitation, prostitution, public intoxication, and menacing. The referring officer believes Carol's legal issues are secondary to her alcohol use. Carol has made previous attempts to address her substance use through treatment episodes and community supports.

Carol grew up in rural Alabama and was raised primarily by her mother. Carol indicates that her father was never an active participant in her life and that her mother had a number of boyfriends. Carol recalls that for most of her adolescent and teenage years, her mother was a chronic alcoholic. She recalls numerous episodes of volatility in the household. Carol is the oldest of four siblings and is the only girl of the family. As the elder child, she felt she was parentified at a young age as she took on the role of caregiver to her younger brothers.

Carol recalls an ongoing physical relationship with one of her mother's boyfriends that began with touching when she was about 10 years old. Carol began experimenting with alcohol as early as age 11. Out of fear, Carol did not disclose the sexual assault to her mother until she was 13 years old, at which time the incidents had escalated from touching to sex. When this information was disclosed, she indicates that her mother was accusatory of her and blamed her for the acts. Carol continued to drink recreationally with friends until she dropped out of school at the age of 16. During this time, her mother was diagnosed with cirrhosis of the liver, and Carol had her first run-in with the law for underage drinking. She was kicked out of the house at this time.

With little to no resources, Carol began exchanging sex for money. In order to engage in this behavior, she would drink until the point of feeling numb. Having lost all communication and connection with her family, she continued in this pattern for many years. After garnering an extensive arrest history, Carol attempts to gain sobriety by engaging in treatment for the alcohol use. She recalls her first attempts at treatment beginning around the age of 24. She does not successfully complete any of the treatment episodes.

Currently, Carol lives in a hotel room, which she has used to engage in prostitution. She was recently physically assaulted and brutally raped during a sex encounter for money. She attempted to address the assault in the way that she knew how, drinking to excess. She reports decreased appetite and some concerns of sadness. Her most recent arrest involved public intoxication and solicitation of a law enforcement officer. Carol did not qualify for drug court, yet her probation officer feels that she might meet success with this treatment attempt. Carol indicates that she often drinks more than she intends, and efforts to decrease drinking have not been successful. Although she has a history of trauma and a current traumatic event, she does not connect her increased drinking with risk. She has few friends and minimal social support. She believes she is beginning to experience conditions similar to those experienced by her mother during her alcohol use.

■ DIAGNOSTIC IMPRESSIONS

Carol is an adult child of an alcoholic. She has a long history of alcohol use beginning in early adolescence. Her use has increased throughout her lifetime and involved risky behavior to include solicitation, prostitution, public intoxication, and menacing. Her behaviors have resulted in criminal charges resulting in prosecution and probation. These behaviors have resulted in this referral to outpatient treatment. Periods of her life are marred by homelessness and current living instability. With continued use, she reports blackouts, restlessness, and nausea. Carol has previous unsuccessful treatment attempts.

She is a childhood survivor of sexual assault and was recently physically and sexually assaulted during a work (prostitution)-related episode. Carol has no history of counseling for her childhood abuse or the current assault. Since the incident, she has increased her alcohol use and is experiencing appetite loss, restlessness, and sadness. Although she does not see a correlation between this incident and her substance use, the issues are likely tied. Carol is experiencing some concurrent symptoms that align with Alcohol Use Disorder and Posttraumatic Stress Disorder (PTSD). When discussing her assault, her presentation is flat and characterized by little to no eye contact with periods that are difficult to hear her.

Although Carol does not present with significant medical concerns, it is important to rule out any medical concerns that would explain the blackouts, restlessness, appetite loss, and nausea. Equally important will be a general medical exam because no care was sought post physical and sexual assault. Carol has limited education, strained family relationships, and lacks a stable support system.

The following are presenting concerns:

 Tolerance to alcohol
 Increased alcohol use
 Blackouts
 Trouble sleeping, restlessness
 Appetite loss
 Sadness
 Engaging in behavior resulting in risk (excessive drinking, criminal activity)
 Intermittent nausea
 Lack of support

■ DIAGNOSTIC CONCLUSIONS

Alcohol Use Disorder, Severe
R/O Posttraumatic Stress Disorder
R/O Unspecified Depressive Disorder
R/O any medical conditions
Additional concerns: Strained family relationship, limited education, gainful employment, and lack of support system.

■ SUGGESTED THERAPEUTIC INTERVENTION

Fully assess readiness to change to identify the stage of change that Carol is in, so that a treatment plan can be developed accordingly. Based on previous unsuccessful treatment episodes, Carol would likely benefit from beginning treatment at Level II.1—intensive outpatient treatment in accordance with the American Society of Addiction Medicine Patient Placement Criteria. Treatment episodes would involve group treatment at a frequency of three times per week and individual sessions weekly. Based on engagement, readiness, and motivation, introduction to community supports are likely—for example, Celebrate Recovery, Alcoholics Anonymous, and so on. As treatment progresses, Carol will be linked with a peer support specialist, who will further add to her support network.

Therapeutic efforts would involve cognitive behavioral therapy (CBT) and motivational interviewing (MI). CBT will be utilized to help Carol learn about maladaptive behavior patterns. Efforts will be made to assist her in identifying her own behaviors along with positive and negative consequences for continued use. Attempts will be made to identify high-risk situations, environments, and triggers for use and developing coping strategies to address these situations along with cravings. Open-ended questions, reflective listening, expressing empathy, developing discrepancy, and rolling with resistance, which are essential to MI, can be utilized to help facilitate the therapeutic relationship and to aid in behavior change. The group therapy environment should allow Carol to normalize her childhood and current experiences while developing additional supports. As she makes treatment gains, the potential for supports can be expanded to a larger community network through Celebrate Recovery, Alcoholics Anonymous, and so on. To enhance potential for long-term sustained recovery, Carol will be matched with a peer support specialist who will help with transition post treatment to aftercare. A minimum of three family sessions will be recommended to facilitate reconnection and integration to the family.

Should PTSD be determined, elements of CBT can be used to identify self-defeating thoughts and to develop counters to these thoughts. This will assist with minimizing and ultimately eliminating pervasive thoughts that do not support her sustained treatment and recovery. Combining these interventions with some aspects of systematic desensitization could help benefit any fears that may be associated with certain environments or situations related to the assault. Pervasive thoughts and fears could be a contributing factor in restlessness, and addressing them could aid in remedying the sleep concern.

A referral for a general medical exam will be facilitated, and follow-up on the results of the exam will be of benefit. The exam can assist to rule out any medical explanation for physical symptoms. The exam can also address the physical and sexual trauma experienced to include testing for sexually transmitted infections and HIV.

A referral for General Educational Development (GED) testing will be provided to address educational limitations. A concurrent referral will be made for job skill training to assist in developing soft skills for marketable employment.

■ FOR YOUR CONSIDERATION

1. Given the chronicity of the issues, which presenting issue would you address first and why?
2. What other theoretical orientations show promise to address the history of this client and the diagnostic impression?
3. What additional therapeutic interventions would you consider using with Carol?

4. With whom would you want to gain consent through releases of information to communicate with on her behalf and why?
5. What additional information do you need that might assist in making a diagnosis?
6. Are there other ASAM PPC-2r levels of care that you would consider for Carol?
7. What stage of change do you think Carol is in, and how would this affect your therapeutic interventions?

Keith

■ HISTORY

Keith, an 8-year-old Caucasian male, came to a community mental health facility through a referral from his adoption agency. An incredibly slender and intelligent boy, Keith appears to be suspicious and angry. He reports that he did not know why he had to go to counseling because he was not crazy. Keith reports having no friends his own age and constantly fights with his brother, who is 1 year younger than him. Keith appears emotionally withdrawn from his adoptive parents and does not go to them for comfort when he is upset. He does things intentionally to distance himself from anyone who shows any care for him. Keith has a flat affect and appears to be quick-tempered, miserable, and anxious. Keith has a history of abandonment and lack of the most basic human needs. He was taken from his biological parents due to the horrific neglect and abuse at 3 years of age that he suffered at the hands of his own parents and grandmother. He was shuffled through five foster homes in 5 years, before finding his "forever" family. Keith has never been diagnosed with a spectrum disorder.

Keith's adoptive parents attribute his symptoms to his disjointed upbringing. They report that his biological parents were on drugs and often left Keith and his brother in the care of his biological father's schizophrenic mother. It was reported that the grandmother locked the boys in a room and tied a rope from the doorknob of that room to another room across the hall so the boys could not get out. The adoptive parents stated that the grandmother would only give the boys a piece of bread and a cup of coffee for the entire day. They were not allowed to leave the room and would relieve themselves in a nearby closet or soil their pants. When this was discovered by neighbors, the boys were sent to foster care. Keith's adoptive parents report that he has little interest in food today, and they make him drink shakes with high nutritional value to sustain him.

The boys were given to a single male foster parent. At one of the foster parent meetings, Keith disclosed that the foster parent was making him take showers with him, and it made him very uncomfortable. This has led his adoptive parents to believe that Keith was sexually abused at this house because Keith refuses to speak of this foster parent or any of his time at this placement. He was swiftly removed from that house and placed with his biological aunt. He loved his aunt and finally felt at ease in this placement. His aunt found out that she was pregnant and could not afford to keep Keith and his brother. She returned them to foster care. Keith was devastated as this was not only hurtful to be returned, but this was his only tie to his family of origin. He was then placed with a couple who owned a trailer park. The boys speak well of this placement, but they were removed when Keith had "an incident" with their dog. There is no additional information on this incident, but it was severe enough for the foster parents to give the boys back to foster care.

The boys were placed with a couple who already had four other foster children. The boys reported that they were verbally abused and neglected at this placement. The adoptive parents indicated that the foster parents would do things to "psychologically terrorize" the boys. Keith stated that this was the most horrific environment that he had lived in since his grandmother's home. Keith talked about this period of time with a great deal of hatred and fire in his eyes. Keith said that they "celebrated" his birthday, got him a cake, several presents, and everyone sang to him. After the song was over, they told him that he could not have any cake and gave his presents to the other foster children. Keith indicated that when his brother forgot his homework, he was made to sleep in the garage in 30° weather with no covers and that he could feel mice walking over him. Keith has trouble with wetting the bed (this behavior goes back to when he was first removed and placed with the single male foster parent). His foster mother would make him strip down naked in the driveway, and she would hose him down with ice-cold water. Keith still wets his pants, and his adoptive parents believe that he can control it because he will urinate a little or a lot depending on his mood. Although almost every horrific detail disclosed involves the foster mother, Keith is incredibly angry with the foster father whom he feels should have protected him.

During the 5-year period of foster care, his biological mother would call him and tell him that she was working on getting him back. She fled with his biological sister when he was originally taken. His sister was 2 years old at the time. He has spent the last 5 years wondering why he was not "good enough" to take with her.

■ DIAGNOSTIC IMPRESSIONS

Keith is entering treatment at the prompting of his adoptive parents and the adoption agency from which he was placed. Keith has Reactive Attachment Disorder (RAD), which is severe and persistent, because the disorder has been present for more than 12 months, and he exhibits all of the symptoms at very high levels. He has been re-homed often and taken from bad to worse placements. He is emotionally withdrawn with caregivers. He does not seek comfort when distressed and is only semiresponsive when his adoptive family reaches out to him. He angers easily, is fearful, and often sad, even when the situation does not warrant such emotions.

Keith has a long history of abuse and neglect. Keith reports that every person who was charged with taking care of him either failed him or abused him. This leaves him mistrustful of others, especially those who appear to care for him.

Keith has a history of enuresis. It is reported that this started with his first foster placement. However, given the denial of restroom facilities by the biological grandmother, this cannot be verified. It is believed that Keith is wetting his pants on purpose when he becomes distressed. He also wets the bed at night and wears "special underpants" at night.

15

Keith is incredibly thin, so much so that his medical provider has called Children's Services to ensure that he is being fed. His adoptive parents ensure that he drinks shakes high in nutrition and monitor his food and drink intake every day. It is likely that Keith has Avoidant/Restrictive Food Intake Disorder fueled by his history of abuse.

■ DIAGNOSTIC CONCLUSIONS

> Reactive Attachment Disorder
> Child Neglect
> Child Psychological Abuse
> R/O Child Sexual Abuse
> Enuresis
> Avoidant/Restrictive Food Intake Disorder

■ SUGGESTED THERAPEUTIC INTERVENTIONS

Treating RAD can involve case management, individual treatment, group counseling, family therapy, parenting classes, and medication. Many foster parents and adoptive parents do not understand RAD. They believe that they are giving the child everything that they have ever dreamed of and do not understand why the child cannot connect to them. One of the worst things that a counselor can suggest is forcing affection on a child who may have an aversion to touch or physical affection. Although it can be very difficult for these parents to understand, their child is not apathetic regarding their relationship. These children simply do not know how to bond with the new parent and may even be fearful of rejection and/or abuse in the new home. Another issue that often comes into play is boundaries. Parents often do not want to place rules and restrictions on a child who has been traumatized and/or neglected. This becomes ineffective rather quickly. Children need limits to ensure predictability and safety. This teaches a child about natural consequences and gives them a semblance of control over themselves. When the child is acting out, a counselor can put together a behavioral chart. Formulate the chart not only with the parent, but also with the child. Have the child draw and color the chart, so they feel that it is their chart. It is important to use positive reinforcement. For example, Keith is hitting his foster brother every day. The goal is to extinguish this behavior. While including Keith, make a chart for the month. Each day that Keith does not hit his brother, he gets a check mark. At the end of the week, if he has seven check marks, he gets a prize. The prize should be something small. It could be an hour of extra electronic time, a delayed bedtime, or so on. At the end of the month, if Keith has 30 check marks, he gets a bigger prize; this could be a meal at McDonalds, a trip to the zoo, or the purchase of a desired toy.

One of the most effective ways to help a child with RAD is by providing family counseling. All members of the family must have realistic expectations. The child's issues will not resolve overnight, and they should celebrate even the smallest victories in an attempt to empower the child toward bigger goals. The family should also be made aware that the child may backslide. Because of excessive fear, it can be incredibly uncomfortable for a child with RAD to change.. This is an opportunity for the family to show the child that they will be there for the child no matter what the challenge. A counselor should plan many therapeutic activities. Activities with the family should be fun because the day-to-day stress can be overwhelming. A counselor should address self-care. If the family is not getting good nutrition and plenty of rest, it can make the work that much harder. Develop a good resource list for the entire family. They may need options for everything from family fun night to respite care. The single best thing that you can do for the child and family is to instill hope. If the child and/or parent constantly focuses on what is going wrong, there will be little to no change. If the family is taught strength-based coping skills that they can use together and individually, it will likely produce a positive result. For example, teaching breathing exercises can be beneficial for the family. A breathing exercise can take place at home, work, school, etc. It does not require money or additional resources. It is a great way to de-escalate many situations. Breathing exercises, guided imagery, and progressive muscle relaxation can be a no-cost way to vastly increase a family's coping skill set.

■ FOR YOUR CONSIDERATION

1. How might this case change if you receive confirmation that Keith had been sexually abused? Reactive Attachment Disorder (RAD) can be seen as a "strong" diagnosis. What steps can you take to ensure that you are not misdiagnosing RAD when it could, in fact, be a behavioral problem or a parenting issue?

2. When we think about nature versus nurture, Keith's problems seem to be environmentally founded. How do you see biology playing a role in this diagnosis?

Carla

■ HISTORY

Carla is a 48-year-old Asian American woman who presents at the emergency room at the local community hospital with complaints of "pain all over." This month Carla has been to the emergency room seven times and in the last year has averaged about 11 visits per month. Despite Carla's repeated visits with medical professionals, she has experienced no relief of her symptoms, which include generalized pain and difficulty sleeping. Carla has had extensive testing of symptoms including magnetic resonance imaging (MRI), computerized axial tomography (CAT) scans, blood work, and other lab workups.

Carla has excessively frequented numerous doctors and hospital emergency rooms without any relief of symptoms.

Carla was born in the United States to parents who emigrated from Malaysia in the 1950s and she is an only child. Her parents were considered "older" when they had Carla, and she was unplanned. Growing up in rural Connecticut, Carla's parents ran their own grocery and its attached bowling alley. Her parents likely had some anxiety or depression. Both of them liked to keep to themselves and when Carla's mom wasn't working at the grocery store she often would isolate and describe herself as "sad" and "unmotivated." Carla's dad also struggled with difficulty in day to day activities and didn't spend much time with the family or others. Probably owing to cultural values, neither parent would seek out intervention.

19

Carla was a quiet child who often felt isolated and lonely. She earned average grades in school. She was accepted at her local community college where she completed minimal requirements for the first year and then dropped out in order to work at her parents' business after her father passed away and her mother was left with the extremely difficult job of running this failing business by herself.

In the late 1980s, Carla's mother sold the business and retired. Carla now lives on her own in the community in which she grew up, and other than just a few "acquaintances" she continues to feel isolated and describes herself as "socially awkward." She states she has always felt anxious in new situations and is someone who is not likely to try something new because of it.

She started working as an assistant for an insurance underwriter a few years ago, and due to fatigue and frequent medical visits she was forced to quit her job. She is currently in the process of applying for disability and is feeling hopeless and uncertain about the future.

■ DIAGNOSTIC IMPRESSIONS

Carla has been admitted numerous times to the hospital for extensive medical workups, to no avail. All of her medical testing has been negative, and the doctors are at a loss regarding the etiology of what Carla describes as "intense pain." Her hospital admissions seem to coincide with increased life stressors. When her father died, Carla presented to the emergency room with extreme joint pain and stayed in the hospital for almost a week. Without any prior mental health diagnosis, Carla does report symptoms that could be related to anxiety and depression. She does mention feeling anxious in social situations and often feels both "physically and emotionally down." She always presents with a blunted affect and seems to be at baseline a slow-moving, morose person who has little hope of improving. Carla has been referred to mental health counseling for pain management in the past and has never followed through.

Carla would likely be diagnosed with Somatic Symptom Disorder, which is characterized by somatic symptoms that can be distressing and very disruptive to daily functioning including work, school, social, and emotional areas.

It is important to rule out any medical conditions or co-occurring conditions such as anxiety and depression that could be contributing to her discomfort. We would note Carla's lack of social support, lack of family support, and the possibility that in her family or culture, mental health problems are stigmatized to the point where she may be responding to stressors with physical complaints. Carla does not appear to be getting secondary gain from hospitalization. In fact, she becomes incredibly anxious when in hospital, and the last few times has wanted to leave against medical advice (AMA). Some of the things that contribute to the doctors concerns include lack of social support, motivation, and some generalized anxiety symptoms when exposed to new things.

■ DIAGNOSTIC CONCLUSIONS

> Somatic Symptom Disorder
> R/O any medical conditions
> R/O anxiety
> R/O Unspecified Depressive Disorder
> Additional concerns: lack of support system and grief at loss
> of father.

■ SUGGESTED THERAPEUTIC INTERVENTIONS

Individual cognitive behavioral therapy (CBT) could be effective with Carla. CBT could help Carla with distorted thoughts—for example, thoughts that dwell on the negative ("I'm never going to fit in or feel better") or self-blame ("I wasn't a good daughter so I deserve pain or I deserve to be lonely"). CBT could be useful with unrealistic beliefs that Carla may be experiencing. Some examples of this may include labeling such as, "I'm stupid and not capable of taking care of myself" or overgeneralization "Nobody believes my pain and everyone is against me."

    CBT can assist with behaviors that prompt health anxiety. Health anxiety includes emotions and thoughts that all feed into anxiety about health. Going to the emergency room and being admitted may feed into the anxiety that something is terribly wrong or that one might be dying. Having medical staff continue to conduct tests may result in anxiety around "nobody knows what's wrong with me so they won't be able to help me feel better." Having fear of the unknown or embarrassment around how you are being treated by medical staff (maybe feeling worried that the staff doesn't believe you or are talking behind your back) may also feed into health anxiety.

In addition to therapy, Carla needs to work with a primary care physician who can be consistent, take her medical concerns seriously, and treat her as needed. It would also be important to have Carla participate in all decision making for both her mental health and medical care. This will help her gain a sense of control.

Carla could benefit from psychoeducation to teach her that physical symptoms can be exacerbated by stress and how to reduce stress responses. Somatic Symptom Disorder can also co-occur with anxiety and depression; so it would be important to screen for both of these.

■ FOR YOUR CONSIDERATION

1. How would you have worked with this family in a culturally competent way to explain the relationship between physical symptoms and stress?
2. What additional therapeutic interventions would you consider using with Carla?
3. Are there any other symptoms or historical facts that you would want to know prior to making a diagnosis?

Todd

■ HISTORY

Todd is a 28-year-old male who is presenting to his general physician after being referred by a neighbor. His neighbor, who is also a close friend, is worried that Todd is isolating and not taking care of himself. Todd used to be seen frequently in his neighborhood. He always said hello to his neighbors and stopped to chat on the way to the mailbox. He was always neatly groomed, made good eye contact, and seemed cheerful. Lately, his neighbor has noticed that he has not been out of his house much, and when his neighbor went over to check on him he noticed Todd had not bathed recently, his house was in need of a good cleaning, and he had not been out to get groceries or basic needs in a while, relying instead on take-out food delivery services.

Todd grew up in the Midwest and has three older sisters. Two have struggled with anxiety and depression over the years. Todd is the youngest by 6 years and at times felt as if he was an "only child." He did well in school and excelled in sports until the sudden death of his father when Todd was 8 years old. Todd's family really struggled with this loss because they were close and his father was the primary breadwinner. After this loss, the family moved away from their middle-class neighborhood into subsidized housing. Todd's grades started to slide, and he dropped out of all sports. He spent a lot of time playing video games and reading and stopped interacting with friends on a regular basis.

Todd's mom, who most of his life was a stay-at-home mom, was forced to start working and found a low-paying retail job. She was eventually moved up to manager at the candle store where she worked, but this resulted in long hours and Todd found himself at home a lot in the evenings and on weekends. His family struggled with the loss of his father but rarely spoke about it, and when Todd brought things up he was told to "get over it" by his older sisters. When Todd is feeling irritable and anxious, his mom sometimes makes comments such as "you are just like your father."

Todd dropped out of high school after his junior year and "hung out" at his mom's. His mom told him he had to get his general educational development (GED) diploma in order to stay, so he did complete it. He took a few credit hours at the local community college in computer programming but found the atmosphere to be too anxiety-provoking. He had difficulty interacting with other students, and in one class he was asked to do a group project that precipitated him dropping out of college. He did find a job at a small upstart computer company where he works by himself at night. The company moved to a different town with the intention of expanding, and Todd decided to relocate with his employer.

Currently, Todd lives by himself. He has moved to a very small community about 400 miles from his hometown. He does not have a lot of friends, other than the few neighbors that he has met. Todd continues to work at night and has found doing daily activities more and more difficult over the past 6 months. He used to be able to shop for groceries for himself but now just the thought of it sets his heart racing and he breaks out in a sweat. In the last few weeks, he has struggled with diarrhea and an overwhelming feeling of fear but is not able to pin down what he is afraid of. At odd times during the night (at work), he finds himself restless to the point of distraction and has difficulty concentrating. Todd has been experiencing difficulty sleeping during the day, despite many years of working the night shift, and he is starting to realize that he is easily fatigued. Several of his coworkers have mentioned that he seems more irritable lately, but he thinks this is probably a result of his increasing fatigue. Todd is so embarrassed about how he has been feeling lately that he is very reluctant to talk to anyone about his condition and finds that staying at home and going to work are about all he can handle right now. He has considered quitting his job so that he "doesn't have to deal with it." Currently, all of his presenting concerns include irritability, difficulty sleeping, easily fatigued, general worry about going places and interacting with others, physical symptoms of sweating and feeling like his heart is pounding when he thinks about daily activities, isolation, and poor hygiene.

■ DIAGNOSTIC CONCLUSIONS

> Generalized Anxiety Disorder
> R/O medical condition explaining symptoms
> R/O depression
> R/O other anxiety disorders
> Additional concerns: lack of social support, isolation, and decreased ability and interest in self-care

■ SUGGESTED THERAPEUTIC INTERVENTIONS

Cognitive behavioral therapy (CBT) could be very helpful for Todd. This would help him focus on thoughts in addition to behaviors. CBT could help him challenge his negative thinking patterns and irrational beliefs that fuel his anxiety. In addition to this treatment, he could consider exposure therapy. Exposure therapy could help him face his fears in a controlled, safe environment to help reduce his anxiety. Group therapy might also be helpful for Todd because he could interact with others and get support from people who are having similar experiences. Todd could also speak with his physician or a psychiatrist to discuss medication options in conjunction to therapy.

■ FOR YOUR CONSIDERATION

1. Research supports medication, and therapy can be helpful in treating generalized anxiety disorder. Would you recommend both for Todd? What if Todd felt strongly against either type of treatment?

2. What other therapeutic interventions would you consider for Todd in addition to CBT and exposure therapy?
3. Do you feel you have enough information about Todd to make a diagnosis and treatment recommendation, or is there additional information that you might find helpful?

John

■ HISTORY

John is a 58-year-old Caucasian male who initially presented to individual counseling in a private practice facility about 2 months ago because of feelings of depression. John reported that his work hours were recently cut, resulting in financial stressors. John has been with his current employer for many years and fears that due to his age and lack of additional workforce training he would be unable to find a job. John reports health issues related to hypertension and obesity. He identifies binge eating as a coping skill, which has negatively affected his health. In a subsequent session, John was referred by the counselor for a medical evaluation and to be assessed for an antidepressant. His physician gave him an antidepressant, citalopram. John was told to continue psychotherapy and to follow up with his physician in a month.

The patient returned to counseling and informed his counselor that he was prescribed an antidepressant. He is currently taking the antidepressant citalopram—a daily dose of 40 milligrams. He also reports that he is taking 80 milligrams valsartan for hypertension control. He has been taking his hypertension medication for the past 6 months. Both prescriptions are prescribed by his primary care physician. John complains that over the past 6 months, he has felt an overall lack of energy and pleasure. He reports that he feels his

27

antidepressant has helped. Prior to the antidepressant, he was unable to get out of bed. John says that he continues to binge eat and eats whatever he can find. He indicated that this morning he ate an entire apple pie before coming to his appointment. In the past 6 weeks, he has gained 15 pounds. John already struggles with obesity—he is 5-foot-10 and weighs 262 pounds. John spoke in the session about how things have just "piled up." In a subsequent counseling session, the patient disclosed that he has been having some problems with his wife. He complains of marital stressors related to intimacy. He states that he is experiencing erectile dysfunction (ED) and that it seems to have gotten worse over the last several weeks. John indicates that he has not been in the mood to have sex and really has no desire for it. John states that this is causing marital discord between him and his wife. The patient denies that intimacy and sexual relations have been a problem in the past for his relationship. He does acknowledge some mild periods of "lack of interest" when he is having increased symptoms of depression. He states that what he is experiencing now is different from that and more significant. John reports significant distress related to this new symptom.

It was recommended that John return to his primary care physician for a follow-up appointment and to assess for potential side effects of his antidepressant medication. In addition, John expresses that he would consider bringing his wife to counseling for couple's sessions while he continues to focus on coping skills for his depression and current stressors.

■ DIAGNOSTIC IMPRESSIONS

Substance/Medication-induced Sexual Dysfunction is the term used to describe various sex-related impairments that result from the use/abuse of drugs, alcohol, or medications. The condition differs from the group of unique mental disorders known as sexual dysfunctions or known collectively as substance/medication-induced disorders (National Institutes of Health [NIH], n.d.). Doctors classify Substance/Medication-induced Sexual Dysfunction according to the specific impairment that occurs in any given case. Although many of the drugs that can trigger the disorder are illegal, an unusually wide range of legal drugs can also potentially trigger sexual problems, even when used according to standard prescription guidelines (NIH, n.d.). The major feature of this diagnosis is a "disturbance in sexual function that has a temporal relationship with substance/medication initiation, dose increase, or substance/medication discontinuation" (American Psychiatric Association [APA], 2013, p. 448).

One of the main features of substance/medication-induced sexual arousal that leads to clinical significance is when there is a development of interpersonal conflicts or difficulties that lead to distress (NIH, n.d.). In the case of John, he reports that his sexual dysfunction has caused a significant amount of marital discord. According to Tufan, Ozten, Isik, and Cerit (2013), multiple sexual adverse effects or in essence sexual dysfunction can be the cause of using psychotropic medication. Approximately 30% of sexual complaints are clinically significant, with the majority from antidepressants being related to orgasm or ejaculation. Issues with desire and erection are also reported, but with less frequency (APA, 2013). However, it is important to note that regardless of prescription medication, depression may be associated with sexual dysfunction as well. Depressive cognitions may interfere with sexual arousal (Tufan et al., 2013). Differentiating between underlying mental health issues and a Substance/Medication-Induced Sexual Dysfunction can be complicated. Balon and Segraves (2008) note how there has been an increase over the last two decades in sexual dysfunction associated with selective serotonin reuptake inhibitor (SSRI) antidepressants. In the case of John, he is taking the SSRI antidepressant citalopram. According to the American Psychiatric Association (2013), the prevalence of Substance/Medication-Induced Sexual Dysfunction is unclear because of underreporting and variance depending on the substance causing the dysfunction. In regard to antidepressants, including SSRIs, approximately 25% to 80% of individuals report sexual side effects. Determining the cause and potential diagnosis is usually related to the relationship between symptoms and medication initiation or dissipation of symptoms with substance/medication discontinuation.

Substance-induced sexual dysfunction is different from primary sexual dysfunction. The sexual dysfunction is occurring from prescription medications or substances taken and not related to any other condition (NIH, n.d.). "The onset of antidepressant-induced sexual dysfunction may be as early as 8 days after the agent is first taken" (APA, 2013, p. 449). It has also been suggested that likelihood of disturbance can increase with age. In this case, John reported no negative side effects related to his hypertension medication that he began 6 months ago. Sexual dysfunction can be due to John's prescription medication for depression because it is a side effect of SSRIs. Should there be evidence that the dysfunction persists after a change in medication, then it may be due to another cause and no longer a diagnosis of Substance/Medication-Induced Sexual Dysfunction (NIH, n.d.).

■ DIAGNOSTIC CONCLUSIONS

> Adjustment Disorder With Depressed Mood
> Citalopram-induced sexual dysfunction with onset after medication use, moderate
> Eating Disorder—Binge Eating Disorder
> Overweight, financial distress, marital discord

■ SUGGESTED THERAPEUTIC INTERVENTIONS

In order to assess for sexual dysfunction and diagnosis, it is very important for the practitioner to adequately assess the underlying cause of the problem because treatment might be handled differently (Pesce, Seidman, & Roose, 2002).

Sexual functioning in general can often be impaired by depressive disorders owing to a loss of pleasure or interest. Therefore, an antidepressant medication can exacerbate the sexual dysfunction. This can lead to the client or patient discontinuing antidepressant treatment because a consequence of Medication-Induced Sexual Dysfunction is medication noncompliance (APA, 2013; Clayton, Kornstein, Prakash, Mallinckrodt, & Wohlreich, 2007). It is important to ask clients about their sexual function in an effort to identify sexual dysfunction early because this is a preventable and treatable side effect of antidepressants and other medications. Otherwise, this can compromise treatment (Werneke, Northey, & Bhugra, 2006).

As commencement of Medication-Induced Sexual Dysfunction is often coupled with medication initiation, discontinuation, or dosage change, the treatment of the sexual dysfunction is often related to a change in dosage or discontinuation of medication (APA, 2013). It is important to work with the client and the physician to determine a timeline of symptoms. If the symptoms are a direct result of the medication, then they may be reduced or eliminated with a change in dose or discontinuation of the medication.

In some cases, sexual dysfunction can be easily treated through a number of different libido-boosting medications such as Viagra. This decision would be up to the medical provider because there may be danger in prescribing this medication in combination with other medications or medical issues. However, these types of medications do not address other potential mental health issues, relationship issues, or life stressors that might be affecting libido, desires, or feelings. In this case, the client may simply be experiencing the side effects of medication (NIH, n.d.). For this reason, it is again important for a counselor to work in conjunction with the medical provider to treat both the physical and mental contributions of symptoms.

To treat John appropriately, his doctor needs to do a complete physical examination and blood work, including testosterone hormone levels that affect one's sex drive (NIH, n.d.). This does not mean that lab tests or a physical examination will show the cause. It is also important to ask about John's cultural, religious, social, and ethnic background, as that too can influence sexual desires and expectations (NIH, n.d.).

John recently began psychotherapy for his depression. Addressing depression symptoms and life stressors may decrease or eliminate his symptoms of sexual dysfunction.

It can also be recommended that John and his wife seek marital counseling for further improvement in their interpersonal relationship. Sex therapy is often recommended for couples that are struggling with sexual issues or intimacy that is not related to organic causes. This may be a potential referral after medication concerns have been addressed/eliminated.

■ FOR YOUR CONSIDERATION

1. What additional information do you need to know in order to feel confident you arrived at the correct diagnosis? What questions do you still have?
2. What specific questions might you ask the client in regard to sexual dysfunction?
3. How might your diagnosis change if the client reported a different timeline? For example, if the sexual dysfunction started prior to the antidepressant initiation? If the symptoms started 2 months after the antidepressant initiation?
4. When might sex therapy be an appropriate referral? Any thoughts about when it might be contraindicated?
5. How important is collateral information in this case? Would you like the client's wife to attend treatment?
6. What if the primary care physician does not agree with your diagnosis? How would you support your conclusions?

■ REFERENCES

American Psychiatric Association. (2013). *Diagnostic and statistical manual of mental disorders* (5th ed.). Arlington, VA: American Psychiatric Publishing.

Balon, R., & Segraves, R. T. (2008). Survey of treatment practices for sexual dysfunction(s) associated with anti-depressants. *Journal of Sex & Marital Therapy, 34*(4), 353–365. doi:10.1080/00926230802096390

Clayton, A., Kornstein, S., Prakash, A., Mallinckrodt, C., & Wohlreich, M. (2007). Changes in sexual functioning associated with duloxetine, escitalopram, and placebo in the treatment of patients with major depressive disorder. *Journal of Sexual Medicine, 4*(4i), 917–929. doi:10.1111/j.1743-6109.2007.00520.x

National Institutes of Health. (n.d.). *Erectile dysfunction.* MedlinePlus (U.S. National Library of Medicine). Retrieved from www.nlm.nih.gov/medlineplus/erectiledysfunction.html

Pesce, V., Seidman, S. N., & Roose, S. P. (2002). Depression, antidepressants and sexual functioning in men. *Sexual and Relationship Therapy, 17,* 281–287

Tufan, A. E., Ozten, E., Isik, S., & Cerit, C. (2013). Discerning the effects of psychopathology and antidepressant treatment on sexual dsyfunction. *International Journal of Psychiatry in Clinical Practice, 17*(3), 223–226. doi:10.3109/13651501.2012.704382

Werneke, U., Northey, S., & Bhugra, D. (2006). Antidepressants and sexual dysfunction. *Acta Psychiatrica Scandinavica, 114*(6), 384–397. doi:10.1111/j.1600-0447.2006.00890.x

Michael

■ HISTORY

Michael is a 15-year-old Caucasian, transgender male (female to male), who is seeking counseling to assist him in beginning testosterone hormone therapy. Michael reports knowing that he was a male from the time he was 7 years old. He said that he always wanted to play with his older brother's toys and refused to dress in anything feminine. Michael preferred to dress in either androgynous or masculine clothing.

Michael first entered counseling at the age of 13 to deal with depression. He reported having frequent suicidal thoughts and a lack of desire to attend school. He also began to withdraw from his friends and spent most of his time at home in his room, often sleeping. Michael's mother became very concerned about him after he told her he was having thoughts of ending his life. It was at this time that she sought professional help.

At 7 years of age, Michael informed his mother that he was a boy and that he wanted to be treated as such. His mother dismissed what he said by "laughing it off" and informing him that this was "just a phase." She would often refer to Michael as being a "tomboy." From time to time, Michael's mother would insist that he wear a dress or other feminine clothing for church, school pictures, and family events. Michael reported feeling very upset when his mother would

33

force him to wear "girl" clothes and stated that he felt like "he was dying inside." As Michael grew older, the battles between him and his mother over clothing became more intense. Michael's parents are divorced, and he rarely saw his father. During the times that he was "forced" to visit with his father, he stated that his father would continually berate him for looking like a "Goddamn boy."

When Michael began to go through puberty, he begged his mother to allow him to take hormone blockers. His mother denied his request, stating that it was too dangerous and that he would most likely grow out of his "obsession with being a boy." Michael reported experiencing extreme symptoms of depression when he began developing breasts. He stated that he tried everything he could to keep them from growing and hide their appearance. Michael also felt hopeless and experienced an increase in suicidal thoughts when he began to menstruate. He indicated that he felt alone and he had no one to talk to about what he was experiencing. He also did not know what was going on with him; he just knew he was different from his peers, and he did not feel like he fit in with anyone. He began to emotionally distance himself from the few friends he had.

Michael's mother grew concerned about his depressed mood and "sullen" behaviors. Her concern was amplified after finding a journal Michael had been keeping, in which he wrote that he hated himself and he wanted to die. Michael's mother confronted him about the writings, and he told her that the world would be better off without a "misfit" like him.

Upon entering counseling, Michael began to deal with his depression and discovered that what he was experiencing had a name—transgender. His mother also engaged in some of the counseling sessions with Michael and began to take what Michael was experiencing seriously. She bought a binder for him to hide his breasts. She also began to allow him to dress in the masculine clothing he picked out. However, his mother continued to deny him access to testosterone treatments because of the unknown potential side effects. She also continued to call him by his birth name. Although his depression had improved, Michael continued to feel invalidated and returned to his feelings of hopelessness. After Michael made a suicide attempt, his mother sought out medical consultation to allow him to begin testosterone therapy and worked with him to legally change his name to Michael.

◼ DIAGNOSTIC IMPRESSIONS

Michael's suicide attempt was the only way he thought he could communicate the depth of his pain and suffering to his mom. He was experiencing Gender Dysphoria in Adolescents. The presence of Gender Dysphoria is evidenced by Michael's explanation that he was a male in a female's body, the desire to be rid of his female characteristics (such as his breasts), menstruation, his female name, and his strong desire to begin testosterone treatments to assist him in physically transitioning into a male. He was experiencing distress in his social and familial relationships, along with an inability to perform in school. Michael identified as a male and wanted to be treated as a male.

He was also experiencing a Major Depressive Disorder, as evidenced by his depressed mood on a near-daily basis, his social isolation, a lack of interest in regular activities, hypersomnia, and suicidal ideation with an attempt. Because Michael's depression was chronic over a period of 2 years, a diagnosis of Persistent Depressive Disorder would be appropriate.

◼ DIAGNOSTIC CONCLUSIONS

> Gender Dysphoria in Adolescents
> Persistent Depressive Disorder, Early Onset, With Intermittent
>   Major Depressive Episodes, Severe
> Parent–Child Relational Problem

◼ SUGGESTED THERAPEUTIC INTERVENTIONS

First and foremost, clinicians working with transgender children and adolescents must educate themselves on transgender issues as a whole, along with the specific population of transgender youth. The transgender population has unique challenges and needs that must be understood and acknowledged in order for clinicians to be effective in working with these individuals. There are many books and articles that have been written on working with the transgender population, along with a wide variety of Internet resources. It is imperative that clinicians are educated about transgender individuals, their challenges, and their needs, long before a transgender client enters the counseling room. One of the best resources for counselors is the American Counseling Association Competencies for Counseling with Transgender Clients (2010).

For working with Michael individually, I would recommend utilizing narrative therapy. Narrative therapy is a strength-based approach that views clients as being the experts of their own lives. According to Constantinides (2012), narrative therapy with transgender clients provides a nonpathologizing perspective and gives control to clients who have been historically marginalized. Narrative therapy can also assist clients in making meaning of their gender identity and can assist them in developing a story of how they would like to be seen in the world.

Family therapy is recommended for Michael and his mom, which would include a psychoeducational component for his mom. Family therapy would include exploring possible feelings Michael's mom might be experiencing after realizing that her child is transgender. According to Mallon and DeCrescenzo (2006), some of these feelings experienced by Michael's mom might include "shock, denial, anger, grief, misplaced guilt, and shame." Michael's mom might also be worried about Michael's safety, health, future employment opportunities, and future romantic relationships. It will be important for Michael and his mother to discuss these emotions and concerns in a safe environment. Part of the psychoeducational piece would include presenting information to Michael's mom on the Family Acceptance Project developed by Dr. Caitlin Ryan. Ryan and Rees (2012) explored parental behaviors that can either hurt or enhance the lives of lesbian, gay, bisexual, transgender, and queer (LGBTQ) children. Their research notes that parental behavior toward their LGBTQ children can have a direct impact on their children's well-being including risk for physical and mental health problems. This research assists parents in understanding the behaviors that increase a child's risk of physical and mental health problems and the behaviors that help promote physical and mental well-being in their child.

36

■ FOR YOUR CONSIDERATION

1. What further information do you need in order to be confident that you arrived at the correct diagnosis?
2. What other interventions do you think would be helpful
   for Michael and/or his mother?
3. What are some other resources you might use to educate
   yourself regarding working with transgender clients?

■ REFERENCES

American Counseling Association. (2010). Competencies for counseling with transgender clients. *Journal of LGBT Issues in Counseling, 4*(3), 135–159.

Constantinides, D. M. (2012). Working with transgender clients: A person-centered
and narrative therapy model. Retrieved from www.goodtherapy.org/therapy-for
-transgender-web-conference.html

Mallon, G. P. & DeCrescenzo, T. (2006). Transgender children and youth: A child welfare
practice perspective. *Child Welfare, 75*(2), 215–241.

Ryan, C., & Rees, R. A. (2012). *Supportive families, healthy children: Helping Latter-Day
Saint families with lesbian, gay, bisexual & transgender children.* San Francisco, CA:
Family Acceptance Project, Marian Wright Edelman Institute, San Francisco State
University. Retrieved from http://familyproject.sfsu.edu

Jamie

■ HISTORY

Jamie is a 14-year-old female who is currently in counseling for assistance with restrictive eating disordered behaviors. She entered treatment with her current counselor almost 2 years ago upon discharge from an inpatient eating disorder treatment center. Jamie has received treatment in patient programs a total of four times, the first two times in a program affiliated with the local children's hospital, and the last two times at a hospital specializing in the treatment of eating disorders in children and adolescents. Jamie was first admitted to treatment when she was 10 years old, the second time was 7 months later, at age 11, and the third time was 6 months later at the age of 12. The fourth time was approximately 1 year later when she was 13 years old. At present, she has been out of inpatient treatment for almost 1 year.

Although Jamie's illness first became severe enough for inpatient treatment when she was 10 years old, she has experienced difficulty eating since she was 10 months old. Jamie's mother attributes this in part to jaw size and bite problems, which are now being corrected with dental procedures including extraction of some adult teeth and orthodontia. She has also received speech therapy services throughout her earlier school years, primarily to address pronunciation challenges

39

occasioned by the dental problems. At this time, Jamie is considerably more verbal and easier to understand than when first entering treatment with her current counselor.

During her last inpatient treatment, Jamie's assessment results indicated that she might also be mildly autistic in addition to having Attention-Deficit/Hyperactivity Disorder (ADHD) and Dyspraxia. She is currently taking 80 milligrams of Strattera daily for the ADHD, which has resulted in better focus and grades at school, as demonstrated by the fact that she is currently on the honor roll in her first semester of high school. For the past several years, she has also been involved in ballet classes, a puppeteering group, and other extracurricular activities, which have aided in the development of muscle coordination and social skills. She uses her Ventolin inhaler for asthma as needed.

In terms of Jamie's immediate family, her mother has been almost entirely responsible for Jamie's care. This is particularly true because Jamie's father is out of town for his employment approximately 50% of the time. This responsibility for Jamie and the other family members, in conjunction with some medical problems, has resulted in Jamie's mother becoming worn down physically and emotionally. According to Jamie's mother, Jamie's father and two older siblings have been diagnosed with "mild Autism." Her older sister frequently displays behavior that is very disruptive to the family. Jamie, her mother, and her brother have all reported that the family environment has improved significantly since the older sister moved out of state to live with relatives after graduating from high school earlier in the year.

Recently, Jamie has again begun to restrict her intake of both food and fluids, resulting in the loss of approximately 5 pounds. Her expressed goal is to stop the eating disordered behaviors, regain the lost weight, and avoid going back to inpatient treatment. While she demonstrates more insight into her own thoughts and feelings, and her health situation, it will be necessary to continue close monitoring of Jamie's weight and orthostatic information (blood pressure and pulse rate) in case she may again need to be admitted to inpatient treatment.

■ DIAGNOSTIC IMPRESSIONS

Jamie continues to struggle with restrictive eating behaviors that seem to be attributable, at least in part, to physiological factors that surfaced when she was only 10 months old. The related symptoms were exacerbated to the point of inpatient admission and treatment at the ages of 10, 11, 12, and 13. Currently, she has been out of inpatient treatment longer than before and seems to have more control over the eating disordered behaviors, as evidenced by her increased intake of food and fluids in response to concerning orthostatic and weight loss information obtained through her weekly check-in with her pediatrician.

It is important to note that there had been a consistently elevated stress level in Jamie's family environment primarily because of emotional outbursts by her older sister. Jamie's mother has also experienced some health challenges, including gastrointestinal problems, that have contributed to a higher level of stress at meal times. As mentioned earlier, the older sister moved out during the previous summer, which has resulted in a significantly lower stress level at home, particularly because Jamie had shared a bedroom with the older sister. Jamie's mother strategized with Jamie and Jamie's counselor to determine ways to reduce the stresses around meal time because of her (the mother's) medical issues. Jamie and her mother report that these strategies have been effective in creating a more relaxed experience at meals. It is possible that this reduction of stress at home may make it more possible for Jamie to successfully reverse the recent downward trend in her eating behaviors and avoid another admission to inpatient treatment.

■ DIAGNOSTIC CONCLUSIONS

Avoidant/Restrictive Food Intake Disorder
Attention-Deficit/Hyperactivity Disorder, predominantly
   hyperactive/impulsive presentation, in partial remission
Asthma
Dyspraxia
Academic or Educational Problem
Sibling Relational Problem

41

■ SUGGESTED THERAPEUTIC INTERVENTIONS

Thus far, Jamie has responded well to cognitive behavioral therapy techniques, including homework regarding eating behaviors and her related thought and emotional processes. Dialectical behavioral therapy self-management skills have also been a focus of treatment, particularly emotional regulation, along with some acceptance and commitment therapy values clarification work. Family therapy has also been conducted with various combinations of family members, and Jamie's mother typically participates in at least part of each session for the purpose of reporting her observations regarding food/fluid intake and weekly check-in information from Jamie's pediatrician.

■ FOR YOUR CONSIDERATION

1. Considering the successful results of Jamie's inpatient treatment, what might be some other approaches or techniques from inpatient treatment that could also be utilized in outpatient treatment? For example, might a group be helpful at some point? How might one be found?

2. While Jamie and her mother have been working with Jamie's counselor to shift responsibility for Jamie's eating behaviors to her from her mother, what would be reasonable goals regarding the complete transfer of accountability for Jamie's eating behaviors to Jamie?

Maria

■ HISTORY

Maria is a 16-year-old female who was brought to counseling by her mother primarily because of behaviors related to school. Since her parents' recent divorce, resulting primarily from her father's alcoholism, Maria had been ditching classes at school and consistently refusing to speak in the classes that she attended. In contrast, Maria's verbal communications at home and when visiting her father had not changed, although she was more irritable than before.

During the intake session, Maria spoke little and so quietly that it was difficult to hear her. This continued in spite of her mother's encouragement of Maria to speak for herself. Over the next few sessions, Maria gradually began to speak more and more clearly, and her mother stayed progressively less in each session. Maria completed homework in observing her self-care and completing an online personality inventory. She also participated in healthy self-calming skill development and worked toward increasing her attendance and verbal participation in class at school. Maria and her mother met with school personnel to make appropriate accommodations in her schedule based on her academic abilities, which they reported as being helpful.

■ DIAGNOSTIC IMPRESSIONS

During the first few sessions, Maria disclosed important information about her fear and anger toward her father for drinking so much that he nearly died from related medical problems. It became clear that Maria's decision to speak only at home and when visiting her father was an expression of feeling powerless to help her father or keep her family together. A significant event in Maria's treatment was when she identified this connection, and then determined that the strategy of speaking selectively was not accomplishing what she wanted it to because it was interfering with her goals related to school and friends.

■ DIAGNOSTIC CONCLUSIONS

> Selective Mutism
> Parent–Child Relational Problem

■ SUGGESTED THERAPEUTIC INTERVENTIONS

Person-centered therapy was used in order to develop an effective working relationship with Jamie, particularly so that she would engage verbally in sessions. Cognitive behavioral therapy and dialectical behavioral therapy were also used to assist Jamie in developing greater self-awareness and healthier self-management in terms of cognition, affect, and behavior. Jamie achieved her goals and was discharged after 10 sessions.

■ FOR YOUR CONSIDERATION

1. How might the diagnosis be different if, in addition to speaking selectively, Jamie were also exhibiting nonsuicidal self-harming behaviors, such as cutting?
2. What additional kinds of symptoms might indicate that a concurrent diagnosis of Adjustment Disorder would be appropriate?

Jessica

■ HISTORY

Jessica is a 15-year-old girl who was referred to your community mental health clinic by the local child advocacy center. A year ago, Jessica disclosed to her cousin that she had been sexually abused by their grandfather from the ages of 8 to 12. Jessica's grandfather passed away last year. While at the funeral, Jessica was asked by an older cousin if the grandfather used to touch Jessica too. After Jessica replied that he had, the older cousin told Jessica she was not the only one. The weeks following the funeral were full of family meetings and various professional appointments, including a forensic interview at the local child advocacy center, to assess the extent of the abuse and number of victims. During that time, it was discovered that the grandfather had molested all of his granddaughters, four in total, and all when they were between the ages of 8 and 12. Jessica has a younger sister, Emma, who was 9 years old at the time of the grandfather's passing. During Jessica's forensic interview, she stated that she felt guilty for "letting it happen" and that, because she had never told, it was her fault the younger granddaughters were abused.

Since disclosing the abuse, Jessica has become more withdrawn from family and friends and is very irritable. Her grades have plummeted, and her parents have become more concerned about her. Recently, Emma discovered that Jessica has started to cut herself on her inner thighs and breasts after walking into their shared room while Jessica was changing. Jessica became very angry and threatened to hurt Emma if Emma told anyone about the cuts. Emma agreed not to tell anyone, but after 3 days, Emma told her mom and dad about Jessica's cuts. Jessica's parents called the child advocacy center for referrals and made an appointment with you the next day. Upon intake, you discover that Jessica has been engaging in self-harming behavior since she learned that her grandfather had molested all of the granddaughters, including Emma. Jessica stated that she does not want to die and does not think about killing herself, but that cutting herself makes her feel better. Jessica stated that cutting herself helps calm her down when she starts thinking about "things." When probed further about what "things" she thinks about, Jessica reported that she blames herself for Emma being molested. Jessica reported that she believes that if she had told someone that her grandfather was molesting her when it was happening to her, then her grandfather would have been in jail and not able to molest Emma. Jessica stated that she also cuts herself when she has flashbacks of the abuse she endured from her grandfather. Jessica reports that there are certain places that she avoids because they make her think about the abuse and her grandfather.

When asked what she thought about engaging in the counseling process, she stated, "Counseling is for crazy people, and I'm not crazy!" After some explanation of how you view counseling and what you think you could help her with, Jessica reluctantly agreed to come back next week. Before leaving your office, you were able to develop a safety plan with Jessica and her mother to help keep Jessica safe until you see her next week. Jessica signed the safety plan, but as she leaves she makes the statement, "I can't promise anything, but I will try."

■ DIAGNOSTIC IMPRESSIONS

Due to the traumatic event and various symptoms, a diagnosis of Posttraumatic Stress Disorder (PTSD) should be considered. Because Jessica disclosed a history of child sexual abuse by her grandfather, there is a clear traumatic event that will be part of the focus of counseling. Some of the concerning symptoms of this case would include Jessica's engagement in self-harming behaviors as a way to cope with her flashbacks of the sexual abuse and excessive guilt she feels about her sister's victimization. Jessica also reported that she avoids various places because they trigger memories of the abuse she endured from her grandfather. These efforts to avoid triggers of the abuse and Jessica's inability to control flashbacks and thoughts of the abuse are clearly distressing to Jessica and should be an area of clinical focus during sessions. Jessica's parents sought out counseling for Jessica because they noticed a change in her behaviors wherein she was more withdrawn, angry, and, now, self-harming since she disclosed about the sexual abuse a year ago. Although the sexual abuse occurred when Jessica was aged 8 to 12, Jessica has expressed more clear symptoms of PTSD over the past year, and thus a delayed expression would be noted.

As Jessica's counseling will be focused on helping her process the traumatic event of child sexual abuse, a diagnosis of Child Sexual Abuse would be appropriate. Not all clinicians may choose to incorporate the diagnosis of Child Sexual Abuse when providing a diagnosis for Jessica. Although it is clearly applicable to Jessica's case, some clinicians would argue that the symptoms are best described by a diagnosis of PTSD and that the diagnosis of Child Sexual Abuse is unnecessary. These clinicians may also argue that it is best to use the least stigmatizing diagnosis possible and to consider the potential harm that a client may come to because of the additional diagnosis (American Counseling Association, 2014). Still other clinicians would argue that including the diagnosis of Child Sexual Abuse helps to create the clearest, most accurate description of the client's experience. Whether the clinician decides to include the diagnosis of Child Sexual Abuse or not, it is an ethical expectation and best practice to discuss the various diagnoses with the client and her parents to review the pros and cons of these diagnoses and allow the client and her parents to be a part of that diagnostic decision-making process (American Counseling Association, 2014). Another diagnostic feature to consider in the case of Jessica is her self-harming behaviors. Jessica reports a history of self-harming and would benefit from specific clinical attention to the behaviors. Although this is a diagnostic feature that may be accounted for within the criteria for PTSD, a clinician may choose to identify this behavior as a separate behavior of clinical concern to be addressed during treatment.

■ DIAGNOSTIC CONCLUSIONS

Posttraumatic Stress Disorder With Delayed Expression
Child Sexual Abuse
Personal History of Self-Harm

■ SUGGESTED THERAPEUTIC INTERVENTIONS

Jessica endured sexual abuse from her grandfather for 4 years; the trauma she endured during this critical period of development greatly affects her sense of self and safe coping strategies. For many children and adolescents, sexual abuse can be confusing to understand and complicated to report. At the age of 8, Jessica and many other children are raised and trained for many years to comply with adult requests, not complain, and do what they are asked. Therefore, sexual abuse is any sexual act that a person may not be able to give consent to (Darkness to Light, 2013). In the case of Jessica, she is a minor and any sexual act between a child and an adult is abuse, just as any sexual act between a child and another child that is forced, bribed, or coerced or involves a developmental age difference of more than 3 years is considered sexual abuse (Darkness to Light, 2013). Sexual abuse includes but is not limited to sexual acts of penetration, force, pain, or even touching and sodomy. If an adult engages in looking at or showing sexual images, shows body parts, or touches self in front of the child, then it is sexual abuse (Darkness to Light, 2013). Jessica has been traumatized by enduring reoccurring sexual abuse and then, upon the loss of her grandfather, was further tormented by learning that her sister had also suffered sexual abuse by her grandfather. The stress, trauma, and guilt Jessica suffered greatly affected her healthy coping skills, leading her to intentionally engage in self-harming behaviors.

Jessica and her female family members are not alone in experiencing sexual abuse; one in seven girls is sexually abused by the age of 18 (Darkness to Light, 2013). Children experiencing childhood sexual abuse have been reported to have a high statistical association for deliberate self-harming behaviors (Romans, Martin, Anderson,

Herbison, & Mullen, 1995). Deliberate self-harming behaviors are associated with significant relational problems within the family of origin, interpersonal mental health problems, and survivors of childhood sexual abuse who endured frequent and intrusive abuse (Romans et al., 1995). Self-harm that involves nonsuicidal self-injury (NSSI) includes but is not limited to a person causing intentional pain and harm to one's body by burning, squeezing, cutting, biting, scratching, or hitting one's self (Washburn, Potthoff, Juzwin, & Styer, 2015). In the case of Jessica, she engages in NSSI through cutting. Approximately 16% to 18% of adolescents report one incident of NSSI as a non–socially acceptable form of coping. Jessica's onset of self-harming behaviors, PTSD, guilt, and the childhood sexual abuse have created demands on her coping that exceed her personal coping resources and available healthy responses (Washburn et al., 2015).

Jessica's mental health and treatment needs require a well-trained counselor in childhood sexual abuse and self-harming behaviors (Czincz & Romano, 2013). Counselors with limited knowledge in evidence-based psychological interventions for childhood sexual abuse need to seek professional training and supervision to provide counseling treatment and services to Jessica (Czincz & Romano, 2013). One evidence-based treatment for children/adolescents of childhood sexual abuse is trauma-focused cognitive behavior therapy (TF-CBT; Cohen, Mannarino, & Deblinger, 2004). TF-CBT uses visualization to address and cope with the intrusive thoughts. An example of how to use visualization while working with Jessica will be provided. The experiential activity of creating stress balls with Jessica will also be illustrated as an example of how clinicians might supplement the development of positive coping skills.

■ SUGGESTED THERAPEUTIC INTERVENTIONS

TF-CBT is a components-based psychosocial treatment model that integrates empowerment, resilience, family therapy theories, cognitive-behavioral, attachment, and humanistic counseling theories (Cohen et al., 2004). TF-CBT is commonly used to treat PTSD symptoms that are characterized by Jessica's intrusive memories and thoughts of the abuse, reminders of her secret and guilt for not telling when she sees her sister, physical reactions, and trauma-related shame (Cohen et al., 2004). In this treatment approach, Jessica will attend 12 to 16 treatment sessions to gradually explore her experience with the trauma and to process her trauma narrative by processing details of her traumatic experiences. The techniques guided by the counselor are to help Jessica directly attend to the traumatic events rather than demonstrating maladaptive avoidance. Counselors are required to attend to Jessica's distress by listening and offering therapeutic techniques that offer an open discussion addressing the trauma.

Stress management and relaxation skills are created to meet the child and family's needs. An example of a stress management skill Jessica's counselor might use is visualization. One helpful visualization for Jessica is to visually see the word *STOP* when negative thoughts and painful memories are experienced. The counselor will process with Jessica memories of the trauma along with her affect, reactions, fears, feelings, and thoughts. As Jessica explores the trauma and her reactions, the counselor will help her process how she has control over the fearful memories by visualizing the fears and thoughts and redirecting her visualization to the bottom of a long pole. The client will describe her fears and how the thoughts affect her as she moves up the pole. The counselor will direct her attention to where she feels the emotional and physical pain in her body. Jessica will process how the intrusive thoughts interfere with her present experiences. As she visually moves up the pole, she will identify how exploring her reactions and experiences in counseling fosters a sense of safety and an ability to stop the intrusive thoughts when they appear painful for her well-being. At this point, the counselor will direct her visualization to the top of the pole to mentally see the word STOP.

This intervention is intended to empower Jessica and help her gain personal strength over the intrusive thoughts and harmful reactions that may be leading to her self-harming behaviors. This process fosters an environment for self-reflection and insight into thoughts and reactions. Once Jessica arrives at STOP, she will benefit from therapeutic opportunities to transition her thoughts to effective and useful outlets of her emotions.

One activity to foster emotional responses is the creation of stress balls. This activity supports her developmental need for movement and manipulation of materials along with therapeutic discussion.

Jessica will be provided with multiple colored balloons to select three colors. She will be asked to select a colored balloon that will be completely hidden and covered by the others. The second balloon will have a small visible section of it, whereas the last balloon will be fully visible. The counselor provides Jessica with options for creating her stress ball by filling a balloon with materials such as rice, beans, and/or flour. Jessica selects the balloon that will not be seen and fills the ball with the selected material to the size of her satisfaction. The filled balloon is tied off and balloon number two is cut off right above where the balloon fills out and the base of the neck. The second balloon is pulled over the filled balloon, with the tie part of the first balloon covered first. The third balloon covers the second balloon by offering a third protective layer. While the client is filling her balloon with material and layering the balloons, the counselor will process with the client her experience with creating the stress ball. The counselor and Jessica will discuss various times that Jessica may use the stress ball to help manage her stress and fears. Here is a list of variations the counselor may consider when engaging clients in this experiential activity:

1. Consider a therapeutic conversation around the color selection of the balloons and the placement (covered, partially covered, and fully visible). The counselor may point out that everyone has various layers of who they trust and process with the client who they identify to be within three layers of trust just like the three layers of balloons.
2. Discuss the challenges when filling the balloon and how filling the balloon is similar to stuffing in feelings and thoughts. Sometimes it can get messy, but the result is a stronger ball—much like exploring emotions helps people become stronger.
3. Discuss how you see the client responding to the filling of the balloon.
4. Consider how the client may find the stress ball useful when feeling _____ [insert whatever feeling you think the client might be experiencing].
5. Associate the balloon coverings of the middle contents to be protectors of the inside. Ask the client how she protects herself, that is, what her strengths are.

TF-CBT is not an appropriate treatment option for clients with other mental health needs that indicate imminent danger for the client such as recent suicide attempts, active substance and drug use, misuse of medications, and severely depressed conditions because these individuals need to receive treatment specific to these mental health concerns (Cohen et al., 2004). Additional reasons to rule out TF-CBT as a treatment option are when other issues take precedence over treatment decisions. A few problems that require treatment before TF-CBT are aggression, disruptive behaviors and defiance, law-breaking behaviors, and harm to others. These problems are best served by directly targeting the condition before treatment with TF-CBT (Cohen et al., 2004).

INTEGRATION OF FAMILY AND SIGNIFICANT OTHERS INTO TREATMENT

Strength of TF-CBT is the collaboration between the parents, client, and counselor, allowing for respectful consideration of the cultural needs and familial preferences (Cohen et al., 2004). In all counseling interactions, parents are the experts regarding their children and are encouraged to advocate for their children's treatment needs within the TF-CBT model (Cohen et al., 2004). Parents and the counselors work in collaboration to assess the child's well-being and coping skills in the home and community environments. The counselor works with the family to explore and educate on healthy sexual boundaries and sexual abuse.

■ FOR YOUR CONSIDERATION

1. How might you determine if Jessica's self-harming behaviors are indicative of suicidal behavior?
2. Many clients who engage in self-harm find it difficult to replace these behaviors with healthier alternatives because the "release" is not the same. Consider ways in which you would help the client explore alternative coping strategies to self-harm.

■ REFERENCES

American Counseling Association. (2014). *ACA code of ethics.* Alexandria, VA: Author.

Cohen, J., Mannarino, A., & Deblinger, E. (2004). Trauma-focused cognitive behavioral therapy for sexually abused children. *Psychiatric Times, 21,* 52–53.

Czincz, J., & Romano, E. (2013). Childhood sexual abuse: Community-based treatment practices and predictors of use of evidence-based practices. *Child and Adolescent Mental Health, 18*(4), 240–246.

Darkness to Light. (2013). Retrieved from www.d2l.org/site/c.4dICIJOkGcISE/b.6035035/k.8258/Prevent_Child_Sexual_Abuse.htm

Romans, S. E., Martin, J. L., Anderson, J. C., Herbison, G. P., & Mullen, P. E. (1995). Sexual abuse in childhood and deliberate self-harm. *The American Journal of Psychiatry, 152*(9), 1336–1342. doi:10.1176/ajp.152.9.1336

Washburn, J. J., Potthoff, L. M., Juzwin, K. R., & Styer, D. M. (2015). Assessing *DSM-5* nonsuicidal self-injury disorder in a clinical sample. *Psychological Assessment, 27*(1), 31–41.

Rhonda

◼ HISTORY

Rhonda is a 28-year-old woman who has been referred to your agency by a local probation officer. Rhonda reported that she has "fired" three counselors in the past and most recently was "kicked out" by her counselor at a local community agency. Rhonda stated that the reason she "fired" her pervious counselors is that they were "clueless and didn't get me." She states that she thinks her most recent counselor "kicked me out because I threatened to kick his ass if he didn't back off." You note that she is smiling as she reports the threat she made to the previous counselor. She then lets you know that she is currently on probation for substance use and her "anger issues."

Rhonda states that she is looking for a counselor who can "handle my past and actually knows how to help me get over it." Rhonda then proceeds to tell you she had 19 surgeries before the age of 10 to resolve a genetic heart defect. She reports that she continues to be under the care of a cardiologist because her heart condition will continue to be an issue throughout her life. Rhonda reports experiencing significant anxiety whenever she drives by a hospital or has to go into a hospital to visit friends.

During the first 10 years of Rhonda's life, she was sexually abused by a neighbor. Rhonda reports that she was also sexually abused by her sister during the same period and continuing until her sister moved away to college. Rhonda was 16 years old when the sexual abuse from her sister stopped. Rhonda disclosed to her mother the abuse she experienced from the neighbor and her sister shortly after the neighbor was charged for sexually abusing another child in the neighborhood. Rhonda's mother stated that she did not believe Rhonda's sister had abused Rhonda because "I'm a good mom and I would know if anything like that was happening under my roof." However, her mom did believe Rhonda's disclosure of sexual abuse by the neighbor, but felt that there was no need to report Rhonda's abuse when the neighbor, who had already being charged for abusing a different child in the neighborhood, would be going to jail in any case. Rhonda states that her relationship with her mother has been "hot and cold" ever since Rhonda disclosed the abuse.

She also reports that she is unsure whether her father is aware of the abuse she endured from the neighbor and her sister; Rhonda never disclosed this information to him directly, but she suspects that her mother would have told him. The family never discussed Rhonda's disclosure of sexual abuse, and Rhonda doesn't know whether anyone ever confronted her older sister about the abuse. To date, Rhonda has never talked with her sister about it, and avoids most family gatherings that she expects her sister will attend. Rhonda states that she regularly gets high if she finds herself at family gatherings that her sister is attending.

Rhonda reports that she continues to have flashbacks of different episodes of abuse. She identifies her heart surgery scars as a trigger. She states that when her scars are touched by anyone, including herself, she gets flashbacks of the sexual abuse by her neighbor because his large hands would brush over her scars when he was fondling her breasts. She also identifies the smell of a particular lotion to be a trigger of the abuse she endured from her sister. She states that she is still unable to tolerate the smell and texture of any lotion and has never bought a bottle of lotion as an adult.

Rhonda is currently unemployed but is looking for a job. She reports that she has a difficult time maintaining employment because she moves around a lot. When asked what causes her to move around a lot, she reports that she has had a few relationships (six in the last year) that did not work out well and that she was living with each of them at the time of the breakups. Rhonda states that she is currently "trying on" being a lesbian because she believes that "women are more understanding than men, so maybe a woman would *get* me better and not leave me." Rhonda reports that she struggles to manage her money or maintain any relationship, stating that "most people in my life end up leaving me."

When asked what she has been working on with previous counselors, Rhonda states that she has been working on different coping skills. In the past, Rhonda would burn herself or get high when her trauma was triggered. She states that she now tries to engage in deep breathing and relaxation techniques, but "they aren't as effective as burning myself." Rhonda does report a history of suicidal ideation, and identifies that she typically will feel suicidal when her romantic relationships are ended by the other person. Although Rhonda reports a history of suicidal ideation, she reports no attempts to take her life.

Rhonda is coming to counseling to be in compliance with her probation. She is currently working on her substance abuse issues with another counseling agency. Rhonda is coming to your agency with the hopes to work on her past sexual trauma. She states that she believes sexual trauma is the root of her anger, relationship problems, and substance abuse issues. She believes that if you can just "make the bad stuff in my past go away" she will be able to get off probation and stay out of trouble.

■ DIAGNOSTIC IMPRESSIONS

Rhonda clearly is a complex individual who has experienced a variety of trauma throughout her life. Rhonda's disclosure of sexual abuse for the first 16 years of life is a significant trauma. She also has experienced trauma from the significant medical interventions to treat her genetic heart defect. Rhonda reports experiencing flashbacks and triggers of both the sexual abuse and her medical treatments, which has created discomfort and anxiety for her. She avoids known triggers like the hospital and lotion when possible and struggles with disparaging thoughts about herself. Rhonda has been very transparent about her anger and struggle with managing her anger appropriately. Based on these symptoms, a diagnosis of Posttraumatic Stress Disorder (PTSD) would be appropriate.

The diagnosis of PTSD is just one piece of the puzzle. Rhonda's symptoms are also indicative of a personality disorder, specifically Borderline Personality Disorder (BPD). Rhonda's pattern of relational strain with a number of significant relationships is one component to attend to when looking at diagnosing her. Some other symptoms addressed by Rhonda in support of a diagnosis of BPD are her impulsive behaviors of substance abuse, self-harming, and report of suicidal ideation. She struggles with her identity as she is currently "trying on being a lesbian" and struggles to manage her emotions effectively.

It should be noted that Rhonda has financial distress because she struggles to maintain a job and moves frequently as a result of her relationship decisions. Relationship issues are a component of the BPD, so you may choose to note the strained interpersonal relationships. Because she is currently on probation, it would be wise to note the legal issues as well.

Considering Rhonda's disclosures about her issues with substance use, it would be important for a clinician to evaluate them and assess their depth. Rhonda stated that the substance use is part of the reason she is currently on probation and that she is already receiving treatment. Because Rhonda disclosed being in treatment for the substance use already, it is imperative that the clinician secure a release of information form from Rhonda so that the clinician can coordinate care with the substance abuse counselor.

■ DIAGNOSTIC CONCLUSIONS

> Posttraumatic Stress Disorder
> Borderline Personality Disorder
> Child Sexual Abuse, Initial Encounter
> Sibling Relational Problem
> Problems Related to Other Legal Circumstances
> Personal History of Self-Harm
> R/O Substance Abuse (not enough information given at this point)

■ SUGGESTED THERAPEUTIC INTERVENTIONS

Rhonda expressed a true desire for a counseling relationship that will promote feelings of safety, understanding, and acceptance.

Counselors providing mental health counseling services for clients of sexual abuse benefit clients by attending training and education on treatment options for counseling the sexual abuse experiences and developmental factors affecting mental, emotional, and cognitive functioning. Given Rhonda's traumatic abuse history, challenged coping skills, suicidal tendency, and feelings of being overwhelmed by the demands in her life, she needs a theory that attends to her past and present unstable emotional and interpersonal challenges and a counselor who is prepared for the predictable turbulent counselor–client relationship. Rhonda may greatly benefit from dialectical behavior therapy (DBT) because this theory was developed by Marsha Linehan to treat individuals who have been diagnosed with BPD and those who had chronic suicide attempts through a therapeutic counseling relationship that fosters self-respect, collaboration, and acceptance (Linehan, 1993a). DBT would provide Rhonda with a team-based approach to treat her symptoms of BPD, emotional regulation challenges, and trauma. DBT is structured to provide four treatment components: skills training for emotional regulation, individual outpatient psychotherapy, telephone consultation or coaching, and peer consultation and supervision for the counselors (Decker & Naugle, 2008). The individual outpatient psychotherapy focuses on factors specific to the client. Rhonda will need a specific treatment for her childhood sexual abuse, need for validation and acceptance, self-harm tendencies, and suicidal ideation (Linehan, 1993b). The skills training component to this treatment approach requires group counseling for Rhonda to address four sets of skills: interpersonal relationships and communication effectiveness, emotional distress tolerance, emotional regulation, and mindfulness (Decker & Naugle, 2008).

DBT offers two stages of treatment to balance Rhonda's emotional reactions and responses. In stage I, Rhonda will participate in treatment that directly works to support acquisition of behavioral and coping skills while addressing and eliminating life-threatening behaviors that reduce the effectiveness of treatment (Decker & Naugle, 2008). As Rhonda develops a balanced response to life stressors and gains the coping skills needed to sustain healthy responses, she will begin exposure treatment. Stage II supports Rhonda's exploration of exposure to the abuse and trauma. This stage will not be experienced until effective coping skills are in place to assist Rhonda in coping with the consequences of being exposed to traumatic life events such as her medical condition, childhood sexual abuse, and family secrets about Rhonda's victimization by her sister. The following treatment considerations are stage I counseling activities:

HOLIDAY DISTRESS TOLERANCE SKILLS

Rhonda expressed that being in situations with others that remind her of past trauma and any contact with her sister induces emotional, mental, and physical distress. A distressful experience for Rhonda may be the holidays, where she needs to acquire useful techniques to accept and tolerate these painful events with family and friends. In counseling, Rhonda will be taught crisis-survival skills when the pain cannot be avoided but needs to be tolerated with mindful actions rather than impulsive, destructive harm (Decker & Naugle, 2008). For an event at which Rhonda might be faced with meeting family and friends that create distressing memories, she will be given a smooth rock that offers soothing emotions when touched and stroked. On the rock, Rhonda will write positive coping skills or positive reminders to support her through these stressful situations. This rock will be kept in her pant pocket to be touched and held when Rhonda mindfully assesses her current emotions to exceed her capacity to self-soothe mentally. Touching the rock will help Rhonda stay grounded in the moment and physical space so that she can assertively communicate her personal needs.

PERSONAL TIME LINE: MY LIFE AS I KNOW IT

Treatment integrating counseling activities to foster exploration of life events may enhance Rhonda's comfort and reduce reactive impulses of deliberate harmful behaviors. One treatment activity may be creating a time line of her life events. Rhonda will be asked to place a line horizontally across the middle of a large sheet of paper. The life-span outline will capture her memory of past events and present emotions.

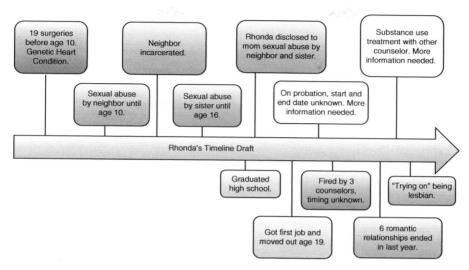

Rhonda will be asked to write and/or draw out symbols to represent experiences she wishes not to share but to represent on the time line.

Life-span outline: Use symbols to represent experiences you wish not to share

- Bottom of line indicates typical experiences across your life span.
- Top of line indicates surprises and unexpected changes, whether positive or challenging.
- List your future expected achievements, accomplishments, events, and traditional life-span developments.

Exploring with Rhonda:

- Discuss her emotions and experiences when creating the time line.
- Explore her coping strategies from one traumatic event to the next.
- Process how she has survived and her personal strengths for surviving.
- Review how she works to mindfully change her relationship choices to enhance her well-being.
- Process what she wishes to work on as treatment progresses.

REFERRAL RESOURCES AND COUNSELOR TRAINING

DBT-Linehan Board of Certification: https://dbt-lbc.org
The Linehan Institute: www.linehaninstitute.org

Homework: DBT provides prescribed homework and treatment for each individual counseling and group counseling sessions.

■ FOR YOUR CONSIDERATION

1. Knowing that Rhonda has threatened her previous counselor, how would you address this and ensure your own personal safety?
2. Rhonda has discussed her mother's response to Rhonda's disclosure. Based on the mother's response, what might be going on for the mother? How might a more empathetic perspective of the mother help you work with Rhonda and heal past attachment injuries?
3. Rhonda is clearly a complicated case. On the basis of the multiple layers, which issue would you choose to address first during your sessions with Rhonda? Why?
4. If you took the past sexual abuse component away from this case and focused only on the surgical trauma, would your diagnosis of this client change? If so, what would the new diagnosis be? Would your treatment strategy change? If so, how?
5. Based on your current state laws and professional ethical code, what are you legally obligated to do in terms of reporting the past child sexual abuse? What are you ethically obligated to do in terms of reporting the past child abuse?

■ REFERENCES

Decker, S. E., & Naugle, A. E. (2008). DBT for sexual abuse survivors: Current status and future directions. *Journal of Behavior Analysis of Offender and Victim Treatment and Prevention, 1*(4), 53–68.

Linehan, M. M. (1993a). *Cognitive-behavioral treatment of borderline personality disorder.* New York, NY: Guilford Press.

Linehan, M. M. (1993b). *Skills training manual for treating borderline personality disorder.* New York, NY: Guilford Press.

CASE TWELVE

Jeremy

■ HISTORY

Jeremy, is a 26-year-old single male, currently living with his mother and his younger sister. At 19 years old, he initially presented for outpatient mental health counseling services requested by his mother, who accompanied him to his first appointment. He agreed to attending counseling if his mother, remained in the room throughout the first interview. During that session, both of them described Jeremy as becoming increasingly depressed over the past 2 years, sleeping 12 to 14 hours a day, and isolating from the rest of the family. Jeremy reported a lack of motivation and problems interacting with his peers socially. He had no close friends and reported most of his energy was invested in writing science fiction and fantasy short stories. From time to time during the interview, Jeremy would connect content being discussed about his own history to details about the lives of fictional characters he developed during episodes of creative writing.

The client and his mother disclosed Jeremy's history with mental health concerns beginning as early as age 3. His mother described him as "a ball of energy" and that he seemed to "have no fear" even when experiencing falls as a toddler. Jeremy's parents were divorced when he was 2 years old, and his problems seem to have been exacerbated when at age 3-and-a-half he went on an extended visit to his father's home. During that time, Jeremy became violent, yelling and biting his step-siblings. His mother reported he was "out of control" for 3 years following unless she was present. Finally, at age 5, Jeremy was admitted to a children's psychiatric facility for several weeks. At that time, Jeremy was diagnosed with Attention-Deficit/Hyperactivity Disorder (ADHD), separation anxiety, and Oppositional Defiant Disorder (ODD). He was prescribed Ritalin, which helped reduce some of his symptoms, and he was then released.

Jeremy continued to experience behavioral problems throughout grade school, including difficulties getting along with other children, following rules, exhibiting hostility toward children and adults. Because of his behavioral concerns, Jeremy was assigned a behavior management (BM) specialist and worked with several different in-school behavioral support staff members throughout grade school. Jeremy's behavior problems caused him having to change schools in seventh grade, after he was expelled for throwing a desk across the room during class. The change in schools appeared to exacerbate his problems, and shortly afterward, Jeremy developed symptoms of Obsessive Compulsive Disorder (OCD). He would become distressed or act out violently if his daily routine was disturbed. Jeremy also began maintaining lists of injustices he perceived himself experiencing, and he kept a journal of his daily activities that he carried with him everywhere. Jeremy was able to maintain a close relationship with his mother, however, and she was often able to communicate with him when his behavior escalated, to soothe and calm him down. He also reported good relationships with his maternal grandparents, whom he often stayed with for extended periods during his childhood.

At the age of 15, while living with his mother and his two sisters, Jeremy was admitted to a local university psychiatric facility for 3 months after having what he called "flashes" of hitting his mother over the head with a hammer and crushing her skull. During this hospital stay, Jeremy was prescribed Abilify, which helped alleviate some of his symptoms. Since his hospitalization at age 15, every 3 to 4 years the same flashes return and Jeremy seeks inpatient psychiatric care out of fear that he may kill his mother.

Jeremy currently lives with his mother. A younger sister also lives in the home and has limited contact with Jeremy; she does not engage him in social activities. Jeremy has one older sister who is married and has a young child. Jeremy expresses affection for his older sister and her family. For the past several years, he has held several different low-paying positions, either in fast food or in retail and has a hard time finding employment. Jeremy usually stays at a single position for about a year before having conflict with management or other employees and being asked to leave or leaving of his own accord. These conflicts usually involve perceived injustices and paranoia centered on supervisors and/or work colleagues.

He tends to seek outpatient counseling services for 6 to 18 months at a time when he is between work positions, because this is when his symptoms exacerbate as he experiences increased paranoia, isolation, and apathy and copes by becoming excessively engrossed in developing characters for his science fiction stories. When his symptoms intensify, Jeremy has trouble separating his own inner thoughts and motivations from his fictional characters and will shift midsentence from discussing himself to discussing a character from his writing. He is open to working with his outpatient counselor whom he has known for many years but does not usually follow through on plans made in session. He responds well to structure and short-term therapeutic goals. However, if Jeremy becomes uncomfortable with content being discussed in therapy, he will excuse himself to use the restroom, returning after several minutes, and then begin discussing his fictional characters and their problems rather than focusing on his own mental health concerns. Jeremy presents with restricted affect and lethargy. He is slightly overweight and has poor judgment. For example, he has made friends in the past with those who were involved in illegal activity or have taken advantage of him financially. When his symptoms become severe, and he is fearful of harming his mother, Jeremy complies with recommendations for inpatient psychiatric care.

■ DIAGNOSTIC IMPRESSIONS

Jeremy presents for counseling services when he finds himself unemployed or when he recognizes his symptoms are intensifying and he fears he may harm his mother. He has a limited support system and relies on his mother almost exclusively for emotional support. Jeremy has been diagnosed with Schizoaffective Disorder, Depressive Type,

Continuous. Jeremy does not meet criteria for Major Depressive Disorder With Psychotic Features because he experiences periods of time, up to a month, when he reports an absence of pervasive depressive symptoms. However, during these times, thoughts related to persecution or delusions associated with his fictional characters remain present. He is slightly overweight due to inactivity and frequent lack of motivation, although when his depression lifts he does attempt to exercise and take better care of himself physically.

Although some of Jeremy's symptoms might be explained by Schizophrenia, a diagnosis of Schizophrenia does not address the severity of his major depressive episodes, and while his previous diagnoses of ADHD, OCD, and ODD include some of the symptoms Jeremy experiences as an adult, they do not include his delusions or pervasive depressive symptoms. Even though Jeremy demonstrated some of the symptoms of an autism disorder during childhood, Autism Spectrum Disorder does not account for his delusions. Jeremy's limited social support and his difficulties maintaining employment are of additional concern.

■ DIAGNOSTIC CONCLUSIONS

> Schizoaffective Disorder, Depressive, Concurrent
> Limited social support, frequent unemployment

■ SUGGESTED THERAPEUTIC INTERVENTIONS

Pharmacotherapy—Jeremy evidences improvement in his social and occupational functioning when he complies with medication therapy to help reduce his symptoms. He should schedule a new medication evaluation so a psychiatrist can determine the effectiveness of his current medication regimen and to make adjustments as needed. Jeremy is usually compliant with taking medications as prescribed, unless his depression and delusions intensify.

Family Therapy—Collaboration with Jeremy's mother will help him follow through on short-term therapeutic goals related to functioning within the home and contributing to the family unit. Involving family will also help Jeremy monitor the severity of his symptoms should hospitalization be required and help him stay on track with his medication.

Bimonthly support group through the local chapter of NAMI—Jeremy experiences loneliness and has little social support aside from his mother. Engaging with other individuals who are managing similar symptoms will help Jeremy establish a support network and hopefully reduce his isolation.

Weekly outpatient mental health counseling—Regular counseling sessions help Jeremy monitor his symptoms and encourage him to develop and achieve short-term goals related to helping his mother with household tasks and obtaining employment.

Ineffective Modalities—those that include abstract or subconscious content such as sand tray therapy or expressive arts counseling. These modalities have been attempted in the past with Jeremy and exacerbated his delusions of persecution, preempting hospitalization for severe paranoia.

■ FOR YOUR CONSIDERATION

1. Consider the many diagnoses that Jeremy had been given since he was 5 years old. What might be the reasons he was assigned these diagnoses? How do you think his developmental stage contributed to his earlier diagnoses?
2. Jeremy struggles with developing long-term goals. If you were to consider one or two long-term goals for Jeremy, what would they be and how would you introduce these potential options to Jeremy?
3. How do you believe family have contributed to Jeremy's problems? If you were working with Jeremy and his mother in session, what do you envision yourself accomplishing?

Dan

■ HISTORY

Dan is a 44-year-old, married father of two children aged 15 and 17 years. He has been married for 19 years and has been employed at his current company for 12 years. He states that his family, friends, and coworkers describe him as a good husband and father: intelligent, thoughtful, dependable, and a good worker. He regularly arrives for sessions at the appointed time and appropriately dressed. Although he is articulate and polite, he often seems somewhat irritable. In addition, he seems guarded. Dan stated that he did not want to attend counseling but was compelled to come to counseling at his wife's insistence.

He states that his wife has been concerned about the amount of time that Dan spends on the computer and his increasing irritability when he is called away from the computer at home. Although he reports that he loves his wife and children, Dan states that he believes that he and a particular famous singer should get married. Dan believes that if the singer met him, she would instantly fall in love with him and would want to be together with him. He states that his wife and children would "be just fine" when he left her for the singer. He further reports that his wife "doesn't understand the chemistry of the love" between him and the singer.

He spends exorbitant amounts of time on the computer looking at the singer's pictures and researching everything about her. The amount of time spent on the computer has prompted his family and friends to begin to worry, especially his wife, from whom he keeps this secret. His wife only knows that Dan spends most of his time on the computer at home and that he is starting to get into trouble at his place of employment for not getting his work done in a timely manner. He reports that he is worried about getting reprimanded again at work.

Dan sent the singer several letters through her fan club and went to see her perform on a few occasions. He reports that he received a letter back from her through the fan club a few years ago; although it was a form letter with a stamped signature, he believes that she sent it directly to him in response to his attempt at contact. A few years ago, he took a flight to where the singer lived and went to her house hoping to see her. He did not knock on the door, but instead just watched the house for a couple of days and then flew back home; he denies doing this again after that one incident and denies intending on doing it again. From that one trip, Dan has pictures of the singer's children that he took from afar with a special camera lens. Although Dan acknowledges that the singer is happily married with children, he states that she would leave her family once she met Dan. He states that his "obsession" has been going on for a few years and that they are "meant to be together."

■ DIAGNOSTIC IMPRESSIONS

The client's primary diagnosis would be Delusional Disorder, Erotomanic Type, because the central theme in Dan's presenting problem involves delusions of being in a relationship (mutually in love) with a famous singer. He denies feeling depressed, sad, or euphoric, but rather states he is waiting patiently for when he and the singer can be together. Apart from the delusions and recently getting reprimanded at work, Dan's functioning is unremarkable. Dan engages in typical activities and behaviors, such as attending school functions for his children; in addition, he reports enjoying household duties and responsibilities, such as cutting the grass and helping clean up after dinner.

Another possible diagnosis might be Narcissistic Personality Disorder, given Dan's idea of "ideal love" and his feelings of being misunderstood; I think this diagnosis is plausible because the client does not appear to consider others' feelings (i.e., his wife's feelings); however, Unspecified Personality Disorder is a more accurate fit as he does not meet the full criteria.

Also, if it is determined that a client has Narcissistic Personality Disorder, counselors would certainly want to address any possible anxiety, depression, low self-esteem, and so forth. Because social relationships with individuals diagnosed with Delusional Disorder and Narcissistic Personality Disorder often suffer in one way or another, therapy for both the client and any associated parties might be beneficial. With that in mind, the final diagnoses would guide therapeutic approaches and goals.

There is a difference between bizarre delusions that cannot occur (e.g., "the trees are walking into my bedroom every night and watch over me while I sleep") and nonbizarre delusions (e.g., "A famous singer will marry me."). While it is highly unlikely that the famous singer will marry Dan, there is the possibility—a 1 in a million chance, but possible.

◼ DIAGNOSTIC CONCLUSIONS

> Delusional Disorder, Erotomanic Type
> Unspecified Personality Disorder
> Other Problem Related to Employment

◼ SUGGESTED THERAPEUTIC INTERVENTIONS

In working with Dan, cognitive behavioral therapy (CBT) is useful to help him refocus and redirect his thinking and behavior (e.g., concerning the object of his affection). Assisting Dan in developing a plan to work around the delusions rather than challenging the delusions is key. Remembering that delusions are typically fixed helps clients function around the delusions. This is critical to helping them live as independently as possible. Mental health professionals do not need to agree with or validate the delusion but rather help the client develop coping skills. With the client's consent, encouraging family therapy (e.g., Dan's wife was affected by the delusions and self-centered, self-involved behavior) will provide more support for the client as they are progressing through the illness. Unfortunately, he refused the idea of family therapy. In addition to family therapy, psychiatric referrals for medication management are essential considering the severity of symptoms.

■ FOR YOUR CONSIDERATION

1. How will you determine whether delusions are bizarre or nonbizarre? Why does this make a difference in diagnosing?
2. Similarities can be found between Delusional Disorders and Obsessive Compulsive Disorders. What are the similarities and differences? How will you differentiate between the two?
3. What would the advantages and disadvantages be of using a reality therapy approach (e.g., Wubbolding's WDEP [wants, direction, evaluation, plan]) with clients who present with symptoms of a delusional disorder?
4. In today's computer-savvy world, do you think that Dan's children might be aware of Dan's behavior on the computer but are not saying anything? How might you broach this delicate topic with Dan?

Tim

■ HISTORY

Tim is a 32-year-old, married father of two children, aged 8 and 5 years. Tim is a software program developer who works freelance for large institutions. He owns and operates his own software development company and is a subcontractor who basically works alone. Tim married his high school sweetheart after he finished college; they bought a home and started their family. Currently, he is estranged from his wife, and she has filed for divorce. Prior to this, from the outside, his life looked like the "typical American dream."

About a year ago, Tim had developed a software program for universities and met with the leadership of a university that was interested in buying his program. The deal would have been a breakthrough for Tim because the university had several branches and affiliates that would also use the software and it would have opened up the possibility of other deals with other universities. However, the university was not interested after his presentation at the meeting, and the deal fell through. After this incident, Tim's symptoms surfaced.

Tim began demonstrating paranoid symptomatology. He became and continues to be suspicious of others and believes people are "out to get him." He believes the university is trying to steal his ideas and his software. He states that the university has bugged his home, his phone, and his computer. He believes that the university is trying to destroy his business and his credibility and has bribed his family members and friends into trying to make him "look crazy." He reports that the university is sending him encrypted messages through the closed captioning on the TV and is trying to take pictures and video of him through his phone and computer. He refuses to share what the messages were, stating, "I will be killed if I tell you." Tim denies hearing voices or seeing things that other people do not see. His affect is appropriate. He reports that he enjoys playing with his children and that he coaches his 8-year-old son's little league team.

After Tim signed an authorization for release of information, Tim's mother reported that he had difficulty interacting with others for most of his life. His career choice was a good one for him because he could work independently. After Tim became suspicious, he refused to work on a computer and closed down his business. He is now having difficulty securing gainful employment and has not worked in several months. His home is in foreclosure.

Although he reports that his wife, friends, and family have repeatedly assured him they are not trying to sabotage his business, Tim states that because of his suspiciousness, his wife eventually became exasperated and moved out, taking the children with her. At that point in time, Tim's symptoms became worse. He states that he began stalking her because he wanted to see her and his children and that he misses being with his children. After one incident when Tim unexpectedly showed up at her house to see the children, his estranged wife became fearful and demanded that he immediately seek treatment or she would contact the police. Arrangements were made for him to be admitted to an inpatient psychiatric hospital.

Upon release from the hospital, he moved in with his mother. He still holds onto the delusion but is able to manage his symptoms and function better, although not at his previous baseline. He reports feeling sad because he lost his business, his wife and children, and his friends. Although he holds firm to his delusions, he states he is hopeful that he can rebuild his relationship with his children and secure employment.

■ DIAGNOSTIC IMPRESSIONS

Many times, functioning in daily life and at work is disrupted by persistent delusions and paranoia. Tim's diagnosis is Delusional

Disorder, Persecutory Type. He demonstrates symptoms that warrant the Delusional Disorder diagnosis, such as believing the university was sending encrypted messages through the closed captioning on the TV and trying to take pictures and video of him through his computer and phone. In Tim's diagnosis of Delusional Disorder, the delusions are mostly nonbizarre—meaning these are things that could happen in real life (e.g., being deceived or conspired against, having ideas and software stolen). However, what makes them delusions is the lack of evidence to support the validity of the beliefs (e.g., family members and friends are caring and supportive and would not sabotage Tim's business or intentionally hurt his well-being).

There is a fine line between Schizophrenia and Tim's diagnosis. He does not meet the criteria for Schizophrenia because he denies experiencing hallucinations. In addition, his affect is appropriate, speech is coherent and logical, and thought processes are organized; apart from the behavior associated directly with the delusions, his behavior is unremarkable. And although decoding messages through closed captioning can be considered symptomatic of Schizophrenia, his symptoms match more closely to a Delusional Disorder.

■ DIAGNOSTIC CONCLUSIONS

> Delusional Disorder, Persecutory Type
> Disruption of Family by Separation or Divorce
> Other Problem Related to Employment

■ SUGGESTED THERAPEUTIC INTERVENTIONS

Most times, delusions are fixed and clients are quite resistant to letting them go. Challenging the delusions or trying to disprove them might make the client distrustful of the counselor and may instigate a power struggle; this inevitably damages the therapeutic relationship and clients might not return, which means they will not get the treatment they need. Although mental health professionals do not need to validate the delusions, they do need to validate the client's experience and feelings. Clients need to be able to function around the delusions.

Helpful treatment includes assisting clients in developing coping skills, decision-making skills, and problem-solving strategies; in addition, behavior modification is beneficial. For example, Tim will use William Glasser's Wise Choice process model when he is thinking about making a decision, such as going to see his children unannounced for an unscheduled visit. In addition, Tim will call his estranged wife each time before he goes to her house to pick up his children for his scheduled visits. He is focusing on his strengths and is streamlining his résumé.

■ FOR YOUR CONSIDERATION

1. Could Tim have had a predisposition that was exacerbated by the rejection from the university (e.g., diathesis-stress model)? How could mental health professionals determine this?

2. Medication is regularly prescribed for people diagnosed with mental health disorders. What would the advantages and disadvantages be for prescribing medications for people diagnosed with a Delusional Disorder?

3. What advantages and disadvantages would group therapy have for people diagnosed with Delusional Disorder, Persecutory Type?

Mike

■ HISTORY

Mike is a 43-year-old, single male. Having never been married, he lives with his mother and receives Social Security's Supplemental Security Income (SSI) benefits. He graduated from high school and has had a few odd jobs doing construction and yard work; however, he has not worked in 15 years. He reports he began drinking a couple of alcoholic beverages twice a week when he was 9 years old and began drinking heavily beginning at the age of 14. He states that he has not been sober for more than a couple of months at a time throughout his life, and these months of sobriety "have been few and far between."

Mike states he spends his days drinking and panhandling for money so that he can buy more alcohol. He states he wakes up during the night and has to drink to "stop the shakes" (i.e., delirium tremens). He admits that drinking consumes his life but states he "does not really see it as a big problem." He reports that his mother has been increasingly concerned about him.

Mike has been arrested 47 times so far this year for public drunkenness, which is a significant increase from his previous arrest record of once or twice per year for public drunkenness. When the police finally put him in jail, he could not understand why he was being incarcerated. The medical staff at the prison helped Mike detox from alcohol and helped him get stabilized on medication. He spent

4 months in jail; the prison staff reports that Mike had some trouble during his incarceration because he did not follow some of the basic rules, such as making his bed. They said it was almost as if he could not remember to do it, rather than him blatantly breaking the rules. They also reported that Mike fell down frequently. Overall, the prison staff described Mike as likeable, kind-hearted, and a "good" inmate.

Within 3 days of his release from jail, he was hospitalized in a psychiatric unit because he was experiencing difficulty with coordination (e.g., walking and getting in and out of a chair) and with memory (e.g., he got lost on the sidewalk in front of his home). Within a week after his release from the unit, he needed to be hospitalized again. Mike was linked with an outpatient treatment facility and was assigned a case manager. A few days after he was released from the hospital, he was arrested for public drunkenness. Fortunately, the police contacted Mike's new case manager and did not put him back in jail. He was placed in a lockdown long-term treatment facility for 6 months and was then transitioned into a group home.

Mike can no longer take care of himself independently. He needs to be reminded to shower and brush his teeth. He is confused about how to operate a washing machine. Although he is pleasant and has an overall good disposition, he has difficulty interacting with others. Mike forgets what is being discussed and begins to make up stories to try to stay in the conversation; unfortunately, the stories have little or nothing to do with the conversation. He rambles and ruminates about irrelevant things (e.g., having to repair the concrete foundation of a home that no longer exists). He demonstrates difficulty staying on task and needs frequent redirection during conversations. His abilities to function and comprehend information are impaired.

■ DIAGNOSTIC IMPRESSIONS

Mike meets criteria for a Substance-Induced Major Neurocognitive Disorder (NCD), as evidenced by his inability to comprehend, hold, and recall new information. He is also easily distracted and has difficulty following conversations. He ruminates and has difficulty finding words to explain himself; he repeatedly talks about having to repair a concrete foundation and has difficulty finding the correct word to denote "house." Although once prompted he will complete simple tasks (e.g., showering), he requires frequent reminders and redirection. He is unable to take care of his finances. His judgment and decision making are impaired. He does not seem to understand consequences, as evidenced by not understanding why he was being incarcerated; he would frequently ask prison staff and other inmates, "Why am I here? Why are you keeping me here? I want to go home." In addition, other residents at the group home have taken advantage of Mike's good nature; for example, at mealtimes, if they tell Mike they are hungry, he will give them his meal. Then later he will forget and tell the staff that he is hungry and missed the meal.

■ DIAGNOSTIC CONCLUSIONS

> Severe Alcohol-Induced Major Neurocognitive Disorder, Amnestic-Confabulatory Type, Persistent
> Alcohol Use Disorder, Severe

■ SUGGESTED THERAPEUTIC INTERVENTIONS

For clients who are diagnosed with an NCD, assisting them to develop coping skills for activities of daily living (ADLs) and independent activities of daily living (IADLs) is a key component in helping them live as independently as possible. For example, some clients do not want to ride the bus because they believe that they will get lost or that other passengers may bully them. In such a situation, counselors would help the client modify behavior—the client needs to ride the bus (his or her only form of transportation), so the counselor helps the client develop a plan to ride the bus (e.g., keep the bus schedule handy, write down specific bus numbers and routes, sit as close to the front as possible, limit conversation).

Mike seldom leaves the group home unattended. Nonetheless, Mike carries a laminated piece of paper in his pocket at all times with his full name, address, and the group home phone number written on it because this is beneficial in helping Mike (or others who are trying to help Mike) find his way back to the group home in case he wanders away. Placing reminder cards in several easily seen locations will help Mike complete tasks such as showering; establishing a routine will also help Mike remember daily tasks. Actively listening to Mike, being fully present, and providing unconditional positive regard is important. Also, focusing on positive things and Mike's qualities is beneficial. One of the most crucial aspects in counseling Mike is validating his feelings, helping him feel cared for, and helping him feel worthy as a person.

■ FOR YOUR CONSIDERATION

1. What are the environmental factors that can help people diagnosed with NCDs stay safe at home and in public?
2. Mike might be feeling lonely in the group home and might be missing his mother. What can mental health professionals do to help Mike with this transition? How could mental health professionals help Mike understand that he may not be able to return to live at his mother's house, especially in light of such a delicate topic?
3. How could mental health professionals help Mike understand that he needs to refrain from drinking?

George

■ HISTORY

George is a 32-year-old Caucasian male who presents at a counseling agency as a condition of court-appointed treatment. During a recent sexual encounter, George demanded that his girlfriend allow him to strangle her until he reached orgasm. When his girlfriend refused, George punched her. As a result, George was ordered by the court to attend 10 sessions of therapy.

When the therapist asks about the assault, George dismisses the assault by stating that she "overexaggerated" the assault and states that his now ex-girlfriend is an "attention-seeking slut." George also states that she is not nearly pretty enough or wealthy enough to accompany him to all the prestigious events that he is "continuously" invited to. He states that he is glad she is gone and knows that there will be many more women "lining up" for a chance to date him.

George alludes to a history of violent sexual encounters. He states that he finds it nearly impossible to achieve sexual arousal without spanking, paddling, or verbally and/or physically degrading his partner. George indicates that he has always engaged in what he refers to as "physical sex" but admits that he has become increasingly violent in the past years. He states that he is now at the point where he must strangle or suffocate his partner in order to achieve orgasm.

George is the only child of a very wealthy upper-class family. He states that he never had a close relationship with his parents because they were very involved in themselves and did not have enough time to focus on him, despite his many accomplishments. George says that he only sees his parents during holidays, but he states that he is not upset by his lack of relationship with his parents because he enjoys his trust fund much more than he ever enjoyed their company.

During the interview, George appears to be arrogant and aloof. He seems irritated and inconvenienced at the prospect of having to attend 10 sessions of therapy. He states that he is much too busy and way too important to devote his time to therapy. He further complains about having to wait 5 minutes before being seen, stating that "he does not wait for anyone." When he notices the therapist's degree hanging on the wall, he scoffs that "anyone can get a degree from a state school." He insists on mentioning that he graduated from an Ivy-League school. George goes as far as to ask that he be transferred to a therapist with a degree from a better school because he does not want to waste his time talking to someone who graduated from such a pitiful institution.

George is currently unemployed. He was discharged from his most recent position as a pharmaceutical sales representative after he failed to make his sales quota several months in a row. George states that he believes that he was fired because his boss was threatened by and jealous of his superior intellect and natural-born talent as a salesman. George is unconcerned about being unemployed because he believes that he will be offered a prestigious position soon, despite the fact that he does not have any résumés out to potential employers, due to his "natural-born ability as a salesperson."

Several times during the interview, George brags about his fancy car, his designer clothes, and his expensive jewelry. He seems preoccupied by material possessions and seems to equate his possessions with power. He states that he has "no use" for people who do not spend money on clothes and cars.

George seems to display little empathy when talking about a friend who recently separated from his wife; George expressed irritation at his friend's late-night phone calls. He stated that his friend should get over the "cow" and stop wasting his time. When asked if he had any feelings of sympathy for his friend, George responded incredulously "Sympathy for him?! He's the one inconveniencing me and he's trying to drag me down with him! He should have sympathy for me!"

George indicates that people have "always been jealous of me" and states that he did not have many friends in high school because everyone envied him. George says that he does not care about having close friends because he has yet to find anyone on "his level." He also states he has been criticized for being too shallow and lacking empathy.

■ DIAGNOSTIC IMPRESSIONS

George was court-ordered for treatment following an assault of his girlfriend who refused to engage in a violent sexual act. The aggressive acts were perpetrated against a nonconsenting adult. He meets criteria for Sexual Sadism, a paraphilic disorder characterized by sexual arousal from psychological and physical suffering of a nonconsenting adult (American Psychiatric Association [APA], 2013). However, in this case, his sexual sadism is comorbid with a personality disorder.

It is likely that Narcissistic Personality Disorder (NPD) is intensifying George's Sexual Sadism. Like many people with NPD, he displays a pervasive pattern of grandiosity, need for admiration, and lack of empathy. This pattern is evident in George's grandiose sense of self-importance and entitlement, perceived sense of success and beauty, elated social status, need for excessive admiration, exploitation of others, lack of empathy, and arrogance (APA, 2013).

■ DIAGNOSTIC CONCLUSIONS

Sexual Sadism
Narcissistic Personality Disorder
Problems related to occupational system (unemployment)
Problems with primary support group (lack of close relationship with parents)
Problems with social support (lack of close friendships, recent breakup)

Problems with legal environment (court-ordered therapy due to assault)

■ SUGGESTED THERAPEUTIC INTERVENTIONS

George, like others diagnosed with Sexual Sadism, may not present for counseling until they are encouraged to do so by an unwilling participant or sexual partner or a court order. Little is known about the prevalence of Sexual Sadism in the general or clinical population; however, most individuals treated in forensic populations are male (APA, 2013). The Severe Sexual Sadism Scale (SSSS) is a useful screening device for forensic populations and may assist with the identification of the disorder. The SSSS consists of 11 items answered yes or no. The item responses are used to code behavioral indicators of sexual offenders who demonstrate symptoms of Sexual Sadism (Mokross, Schilling, Eher, & Nitschke, 2012).

Prognosis and participation in treatment may be dependent on client motivation (i.e., clients experiencing symptoms as problematic and desiring change may be more motivated). The treatment success of paraphilic disorders depends on the duration, frequency, and severity of the symptoms. Cognitive behavioral therapy (CBT) is recommended to decrease sexual urges, teach coping skills, identify triggers, and redirect inappropriate behaviors to more socially acceptable behaviors (APA, 2013).

A single treatment strategy has not been proven superior or reliable with clients with NPD. To date, none have been empirically tested for evidence of efficacy (Ronningstam, 2015). Despite limited treatment data, a strong therapeutic alliance is positively correlated with successful treatment of individuals diagnosed with a personality disorder. The alliance can be strengthened with the NPD population through the identification of specific treatment goals and target behaviors that are agreed on by both the client and clinician. Given the focus on specific behaviors and concrete goals, CBT is recommended for use with personality disorders including NPD. The focus is placed on educating the client about problem behaviors, validating the client, and identifying target behaviors that are problematic. CBT strategies can also be used to identify and replace cognitive distortions and thinking that perpetuate the primary diagnostic features of NPD—grandiosity, need for admiration, and lack of empathy (Ronningstam, 2014).

■ FOR YOUR CONSIDERATION

1. How might your diagnosis change if George was having sexual fantasies about a minor?
2. What information do you feel you still need to know in order to feel confident that you arrived at the correct diagnosis?
3. How might your diagnosis change if George's symptoms and behaviors were limited to consensual sadomasochistic role-play?
4. How is George's diagnosis of NPD intensifying his diagnosis of Sexual Sadism?

■ REFERENCES

American Psychiatric Association. (2013). *Diagnostic and statistical manual of mental disorders* (5th ed.). Arlington, VA: American Psychiatric Publishing.

Mokross, A., Schilling, F., Eher, R., & Nitschke, J. (2012). The severe sexual sadism scale: Cross-validation and scale properties. *Psychological Assessment, 24,* 764–769.

Ronningstam, E. (2011). Narcissistic personality disorder. *Personality and Mental Health, 5,* 222–227.

Ronningstam, E. F. (2014). Narcissistic personality disorder. In G. O. Gabbard (Ed.), *Gabbard's treatments of psychiatric disorders* (5th ed., pp. 1073–1086). Arlington, VA: American Psychiatric Publishing.

Jonathan

■ HISTORY

Jonathan is a 19-year-old college freshman who currently lives with his mother and his 21-year-old sister—when she is home from college. Jonathan presented in a depressed mood with a congruent affect. He agreed to attend counseling at the suggestion of his mother. Jonathan identifies as a good student in high school who graduated with a 4.0 grade point average, the completion of four college courses before graduation, and the recipient of multiple scholarships and academic awards. Jonathan reported being very focused in high school even to the exclusion of a social life. He is in good physical condition and reportedly holds multiple high school records in track and field. Jonathan reports an ongoing focus with physical fitness and attending the gym multiple times per week. Jonathan presented because he is having difficulty after leaving college after only 3 weeks. Jonathan explains that he knew that it would be hard but that he was not prepared for how much work it would require. Jonathan described having difficulty keeping up with the readings and putting as much effort as is required to perform in the manner in which he had in high school. He expressed feeling overwhelmed with fitting everything in and simply could not handle it any longer. Jonathan reports that he feels like a failure and that he does not think that he is smart enough to attend college.

Jonathan described a difficult childhood during which his mom and dad divorced. He identifies his relationship with his father as "not close" and indicated that his dad was controlling and emotionally abusive. Jonathan's father is very religious and holds very black-and-white beliefs about living a "moral" life. Jonathan reported a close relationship with his mother growing up—she had primary custody and Jonathan would visit his father every other weekend. Jonathan reports believing that it was his moral obligation to do his best in whatever he does. Jonathan described a history of worrying about school dating back to the fifth grade where he became focused on his future academic success. He reported that it became apparent to him that he spent considerably more time on his schoolwork than his academically comparable peers while still in high school. Jonathan reports that his need to work harder and longer than his peers means that he is just not as smart as them. He reports a history of becoming restless and irritable and having difficulty sleeping, especially before exams. In order to manage the worry, he would study and review material constantly, often not getting much more than 5 hours of sleep a night. Jonathan reported feeling nervous and unsettled when he did not fill his downtime with productive work, making it difficult to engage with peers in social activities.

Upon returning from college and per his mother's insistence, Jonathan returned to a job at a local restaurant that he had during high school. Jonathan discussed working at the restaurant and expressed his frustration with coworkers and how they do not seem to care about the vision that the CEO has for the company. He discussed having difficulty being as productive as his coworkers because it often takes him longer to perform certain tasks to the standards that he believes are required. He fears that he will be fired if he cannot perform the tasks to the standards that are dictated by the employee handbook. Jonathan appeared confused when asked if he liked his job or to identify times that he enjoyed his job. He maintains that he likes his job because he knows exactly what is expected of him but that he would not say that it is enjoyable. Jonathan reported that making friends at work is difficult because there really is not time for socializing. Although his coworkers frequently socialize, it is not really permitted and there are always other job duties that require attention. Jonathan reports that he and his mother have gotten into arguments lately because she offers "wisdom" that is not helpful. Jonathan's mother frequently tells him to relax and reminds him that he is not at school so he should be less anxious and stressed.

Jonathan had difficulty identifying times that he was able to enjoy himself without worry or fear that he would do or say something wrong. Jonathan expresses concern that others will get the wrong impression and draw conclusions about him that are not true. Throughout the initial session, Jonathan frequently apologized for "getting off topic," for believing that he did not answer questions correctly and for taking up so much time filling out paperwork. Jonathan had difficulty completing the *DSM-5* Cross-Cutting Symptom Measure, continually asking questions for clarification and reporting that he did not want to give the wrong impression stating that he knows how important the paperwork is to his treatment. Jonathan discussed some friendships that he had in high school but reported that they were mainly individuals with whom he had classes and their interactions almost always involved course work. Jonathan identifies with his friends through his academic success and fears that his friends will no longer like him because of his recent academic "failure." Jonathan reports that he goes from being irritable, restless, and having frequent headaches to being completely exhausted. At times he is so tired that he does not have the energy to go to the gym. Despite feeling exhausted, he reports that he often has difficulty falling asleep at night because he is consumed by thoughts about what he has not done, what he needs to do, and what he could or should have done better. Most mornings he wakes up feeling "on edge," as if something is about to happen. Jonathan reports that he wants to go back to school next fall and that he would like to figure out how to relax and have more fun in life.

■ DIAGNOSTIC IMPRESSIONS

Jonathan describes excessive anxiety and apprehensive expectation occurring more days than not for at least 6 months. Jonathan experienced some relief by overfunctioning throughout high school but was unable to continue with his coping mechanism when the workload increased in college. Despite overfunctioning, Jonathan was unable to control the worrying to any great extent, often experiencing restlessness, irritability, muscle tension (headaches), fatigue, and difficulty falling asleep. Jonathan's worry appears to be focused on his competence and the quality of his performance. Jonathan's worries are excessive and interfere significantly with academic functioning, work, and social/peer relationships that have a negative effect on his quality of life.

Jonathan demonstrates some insight regarding his anxiety—understanding that he cannot continue as he has been if he wants to not only manage but enjoy his life. However, he adamantly argues that his success in high school can only be attributed to the excessive amount of attention he gave to his course work. Jonathan demonstrates a desire to do things the "right" way and believes that all matters in life should be given great value and addressed in the same manner.

■ DIAGNOSTIC CONCLUSION

Generalized Anxiety Disorder

■ SUGGESTED THERAPEUTIC INTERVENTIONS

Pharmacotherapy—Jonathan should schedule an evaluation with a psychiatrist to assess the appropriateness of medication to reduce his anxious symptoms.

Individual Therapy—Individual weekly sessions to work toward Jonathan's self-identified goal to return to college, be less stressed, and find more fun in life. The use of cognitive behavior therapy (CBT) has been well established as an evidence-based treatment for Generalized Anxiety Disorder. Jonathan should develop a working knowledge of the cognitive, behavioral, and physiological elements of anxiety. He will also benefit from understanding the role that his negative automatic thoughts (overestimates probability of negative outcomes and underestimates his own ability) contribute to his anxiety.

■ FOR YOUR CONSIDERATION

1. What other information would you like to know in determining the best course of treatment for Jonathan?

2. What contributing factors do you believe have influenced Jonathan's diagnosis of Generalized Anxiety Disorder?
3. Why do you think it took Jonathan until this stage in his development to seek help?
4. Would you screen Jonathan for any other diagnoses? If so, which ones? Why?
5. What role do you believe the development of self-esteem plays in the evolution of an anxiety disorder?

Julia

■ HISTORY

Julia is an 8-year-old female who lives with her mother, father, and 5-year-old brother. Julia presented with her mother and brother for her initial visit due to concerns that had become more pronounced as her school career progressed. Julia's father travels frequently for work and was not able to attend counseling sessions. Julia is in the second grade at a public elementary school in a suburban neighborhood.

Julia presented in a pleasant and talkative mood. Julia was very animated, exploring the room, touching, picking up objects, and often interrupting her mom by putting the objects in her face. Julia did not sit down for the duration of the initial session and moved from task to task without engaging in any one activity for more than a few minutes. Julia had to be reminded multiple times not to climb on the couch. Julia frequently intruded on her brother's play by grabbing objects from him and whined to her mom when he did not cooperate with her intrusion by saying that he would not "share." At times, Julia would intrude on her brother's play by giving him directions on what to do and how to play.

During the initial session, her mom reported that Julia has always demonstrated difficulty following directions and completing various tasks at home. Her mom specifically reported that cleaning her room has become a constant battle because Julia will remain in her room for hours, often "playing" when she should be cleaning. Her mom reports that she is often frustrated because Julia does not listen to her even when she is speaking directly to her. Her mom admits that Julia knows how to clean her room and can do so with constant supervision and specific instructions—what to do when—but states that they (parents) refuse to "overfunction" for their daughter who is "old enough" to complete independent chores. Her mom states that if Julia was more organized she would not have such a big mess to tackle in her room. Her mom also states that Julia often becomes overly emotional with "things that really aren't a big deal." For example, she can become tearful when she is not going to a place she likes to eat or when her brother plays with something that is hers and she is afraid that he will break it. Her mom described a situation in which Julia was upset because she could not wear a shirt that she had outgrown, and it took her 20 minutes to calm down and stop crying.

Her mom reports that Julia has been constantly "on the go" since she could walk. Julia rarely sits still and constantly has something to say. Her mom explained that they stopped going out to restaurants when Julia was a toddler because she could not sit still and would disrupt the entire restaurant. Her mom reports constantly having to tell Julia to "sit like a lady" and that she gave up on dresses long ago because Julia is constantly climbing on objects or sprawling around on the floor. Julia's mom explains having difficulty getting anything done when Julia was little because her daughter would not remain engaged in any activity long enough.

Her mom reports that there have been additional problems as Julia has gotten older and the demands of school have increased. Based on teacher reports, Julia has difficulty remaining in her seat and following the directions of the classroom as well as specific directions from her teachers. Julia has difficulty completing her seatwork, often playing with items in her desk and attempting to engage other students or simply staring off into space. Her mom reports that getting Julia to complete her homework is a nightly struggle that takes hours to finish. Despite finishing her homework, Julia often loses homework points because she frequently fails to follow her morning routine at school and forgets to turn it in. Julia's teacher reports that she has to constantly remind Julia to raise her hand if she wants to answer a question or needs to get the teacher's attention. Another area of concern for the school is Julia's difficulty with walking and/or waiting in line—she often gets out of line to talk to peers and has difficulty keeping her hands to herself. Julia also displays some intrusive behaviors with peers, often interrupting games and taking others' belongings without asking. Her mom believes that these intrusive and impulsive behaviors have made it difficult for Julia to make and maintain friendships. Her mom reports that Julia has the habit of being too honest by saying whatever comes to her mind without considering others' feelings. Despite the various concerns in the school setting, Julia's teachers report that when she pays attention she avoids careless mistakes and generally knows the material. All parties involved agree that Julia is a bright girl.

Julia reports that her parents are always yelling at her and that she is always getting in trouble. Julia maintains that she wants to do well in school but reports that the teachers hate her and make her work more difficult on purpose. Julia expressed sadness and frustration at not having any close friends and reported that she tries to play with the girls at recess but that they always run away from her.

■ DIAGNOSTIC IMPRESSIONS

According to her mother's report, Julia has demonstrated a persistent pattern of inattention, hyperactivity, and impulsivity since she was a toddler. Julia's symptoms include making careless mistakes in schoolwork, difficulty sustaining attention/focus during tasks, does not seem to listen when spoken to directly, often does not follow through on instructions, fails to finish schoolwork and chores, demonstrates difficulty organizing tasks and activities, is easily distracted by extraneous stimuli, is often forgetful in daily activities, often squirms in her seat, leaves her seat when expected to remain, runs and climbs in situations where it is inappropriate, is unable to play or engage in leisure activities quietly, is often "on the go," talks excessively, blurts out answers, has difficulty awaiting her turn, and often interrupts or intrudes on others. The difficulties that Julia is experiencing have demonstrated a greater impact as academic expectations and the expectation of independence have increased. Julia's symptoms have persisted for at least 6 months, have had a direct negative impact on social and academic functioning, and are present in two or more settings (home and school).

97

■ DIAGNOSTIC CONCLUSIONS

Attention-Deficit/Hyperactivity Disorder, Combined Presentation, Moderate

■ SUGGESTED THERAPEUTIC INTERVENTIONS

Pharmacotherapy—Julia's mother should schedule an evaluation with a psychiatrist to assess the appropriateness of Attention-Deficit/Hyperactivity Disorder (ADHD) medication to reduce her symptoms.

Family/Individual Therapy—Individual sessions with parents to educate the parents about the symptoms, causes, and treatments of ADHD. Individual sessions will also be used to teach behavior management skills to increase prosocial behaviors and decrease disruptive behaviors coupled with family sessions (with Julia) to model and reinforce positive parent–child interactions.

School Collaboration—Therapist should assist the parents in collaborating with the school to develop a behavioral management system in the classroom to reinforce appropriate behavior and to improve school performance. In order to increase communication between the school and home, a communication system should be established (i.e., daily behavior reports).

Social/Peer Relationship Building—Involvement in a child-based group program that focuses on peer relationships will assist Julia in developing and maintaining appropriate friendships. The program should not occur without simultaneous parent behavior management training and ongoing collaboration with the program instructors.

■ FOR YOUR CONSIDERATION

1. What other information would you like to know in determining the best course of treatment for Julia?
2. How do the family dynamics presented contribute to Julia's difficulties?

Cate

■ HISTORY

Cate is a 33-year-old divorced female who lives in her own apartment in a midsize city with her 16-year-old daughter, 4-year-old daughter, and 18-week-old daughter. Cate has a master's degree in her field and has worked for the same company since her internship in graduate school 9 years ago and has received regular promotions and management opportunities. Cate states that she enjoys her current job and likes her coworkers, but she has recently changed supervisors, from a female that she had since her start date to a male from a different location within the company. She states that her new supervisor "hates her" because he knew that her former supervisor recommended her for the position. She fears termination because of this. Cate states that she did not apply for the position because she was newly pregnant but did not announce it yet to the company and thought that it would "look bad" if she took the job and then went on maternity leave.

Cate is heterosexual and is not involved in a current romantic relationship. She was married for 10 years and divorced last year, although she had been separated from her husband for the past 4 years. Her younger two children are fathered by her ex-boyfriend, the person she cheated on her husband with; however, she had recently broken up with him due to repeated physical and emotional abuse. The last time she saw her ex-boyfriend, he had thrown her into a wall while she was pregnant and her daughters were watching. The 16-year-old called the police, and charges were pressed against the ex-boyfriend.

Cate states that she has been having mental health symptoms for several years. She states that she had been diagnosed with anxiety and fears being alone. When asked to describe her symptoms, she states that they began when she was an adolescent and includes difficulty concentrating, impulsivity, and strained relationships. She falls in and out of romantic relationships easily, and most of those relationships are turbulent. Her most secure relationship was with her husband, but she could not take the "dullness of marriage" and had multiple affairs. The last affair leading to a pregnancy led her husband to separate. She noted that he wanted to try marriage counseling and pretend the baby was his, but she "couldn't live a lie."

Cate noted that her mother has a history of depression and her father has Posttraumatic Stress Disorder (PTSD) as a result of his combat experience in the Vietnam War. Cate said that her older sister probably has Obsessive Compulsive Disorder, and when pressed about her sister's symptoms, Cate said that her older sister must have things "just so" and likes to control the situation. Cate denies suicidal ideation, homicidal ideation, and audio or visual hallucinations and can contract for safety.

Cate's father served two tours in the Army in Vietnam. During the second tour, he was ambushed by the Vietcong while on a patrol and severely injured his back and arm. He was rehabilitated but often had flashbacks of the ambush and a "friendly fire" air raid resulting from misinterpreted coordinates. Cate said that as children, she and her sister Brynn would be awakened by their father pulling them out of bed and screaming "Air Raid!" at them and instructing them to hide under the bed. Once, when Cate was about 8 years old and her sister 10, Brynn tried to get him to snap out of it and their father punched her so hard that she was knocked unconscious. Cate tried to run to get their mother but she was tackled to the ground by her father and asked, "Do you want to get yourself killed?" Cate said her father kept her pinned down, half under the bed, half out, for the rest of the night. She said that she must have fallen asleep or passed out because she does not remember what had happened. In the morning, she awoke to the sound of Brynn crying in the kitchen as their mother put an ice pack on Brynn's face. Their mother insisted that

Brynn "fell" and made the girls promise to tell everyone that story if asked. They were told that if they deviated from the "Brynn fell" script, they would be taken away and would live somewhere else.

Cate said that was not the first or most traumatic incident caused by her father's PTSD. Her most traumatic memory was when she was 5 years old. Cate said that her father was giving her a bath and they were laughing and singing the "Rubber Ducky" song from Sesame Street. She said that she took her duck and dropped it in the water with a lot of force, causing a large splash. Her father went silent, and she said that his "eyes went dead." The next thing she knew, her head was held underwater and he was whispering intently, "Hide, hide! They are coming!" She said that she remembers struggling to get air and that she could not slip from his grasp. She remembers how desperate she felt but said that there was a release and then she passed out. Cate found out later that Brynn walked by when she heard the splashing and started screaming for their mother. Her mother said that she came into the bathroom and flicked the lights on and off. Somehow that flicking, according to Cate's mother, brought him back. He got up and walked out of the bathroom and never gave the girls a bath again.

Cate does not give her children baths. She showers with them when they are babies or toddlers, and when married, she had her ex-husband bathe the children. One of the chores of her oldest daughter is to bathe her sisters. Cate is not afraid that she will hold them under the water, but she fears what would happen if they drowned. She does not want them to feel the panic that she felt that day.

Cate has used marijuana since she was 12 years old, except when she was pregnant or nursing. She said that she has some friends who like to smoke, and she often smokes a joint or two with her friends and purchases it directly from her friends, but it has not progressed to the point where she will actually go and seek out marijuana from a dealer. It is more of a "if it is there, I will smoke it."

Cate uses substances, particularly marijuana, to numb herself so that she does not feel intense emotions and anxiety. They were her "coping mechanism that always seems to work"—at least for a short period of time. She reports that she often feels anxious, like she "needs to jump out of" her skin, and that marijuana mellows her out and enables her to "be a chill mom." However, Cate

101

is concerned that her company will drug-test employees now that they are contracting with other firms to provide services on a consultation basis.

In addition, Cate is financially reckless. During her graduate school years, she took out the maximum amount of student loans, even though she had a full tuition scholarship and a husband who supported her financially. She does not recall what she purchased with that money, but she gave some of it away to her various lovers. When she and her husband separated, she found herself in a mountain of debt, and "her credit is shot," despite making nearly six figures per year. She often "forgets" to pay her bills and has had her electricity shut off multiple times. Her mother recently made her a budget and has her bills being paid through automatic deductions so that this does not happen again.

Cate is intelligent and, professionally she is quite successful. Her mother is her biggest support and helps Cate whenever she can. Cate reports that she can always count on Brynn when she needs something, but they are not very close. Cate reports that her children are well adjusted. Her ex-husband serves as a father figure for her two older children and often takes all of them out to dinner, ice-skating, or other events. She reports that their relationship is actually quite good, and he is now her "best friend."

■ DIAGNOSTIC IMPRESSIONS

Cate demonstrates the residual effects of childhood trauma on a person's life. On the surface, Cate is an attractive, educated, professional mother who seems to have her life in order. However, the trauma that she experienced as a result of having a father who was also traumatized has stayed with her, manifesting in various problems with substances and sexual and financial impulsivity and damaging relationships.

Cate self-medicates her anxiety through cannabis use. Although she does not seek out dealers for her own supply of marijuana, she surrounds herself with people so that she can readily smoke when she feels the need. Unfortunately, her use of cannabis may lead to employment woes if her company decides to drug-test.

Cate lacks positive coping skills, and to date, substance use and romantic relationships are her way of coping. It will be a challenge to teach her new coping skills and have her master their application. Cate has many symptoms of Borderline Personality Disorder.

■ DIAGNOSTIC CONCLUSIONS

Cannabis Use Disorder, Moderate
Borderline Personality Disorder
Personal History (Past History) of Spouse or Partner Violence, Physical
Other Personal History of Psychological Trauma

■ SUGGESTED THERAPEUTIC INTERVENTIONS

Dialectical Behavior Therapy—Cate displays many symptoms of Borderline Personality Disorder. Given that dialectical behavioral therapy is the only evidence-based treatment for Borderline Personality Disorder, this therapeutic approach should be used so that Cate may learn distress tolerance skills and how to regulate her emotions without cannabis. These skills may prove helpful to managing Cate's symptoms.

Narcotics Anonymous (NA)—Cate might find it beneficial to attend NA groups so that she can work through her need to use cannabis as a way to self-medicate and cope with stressors. Having others who are in recovery and using NA as a support system may assist Cate in developing new, healthy relationships.

■ FOR YOUR CONSIDERATION

1. Cate's early childhood traumas have greatly affected her life and still do to this day. What other treatment recommendations would you make for Cate?
2. How is Borderline Personality Disorder related to trauma and addiction?
3. Given what Cate and Brynn have been through together, why do you think they are not close even though Brynn is always there if Cate needs her?

Alec

■ HISTORY

Alec is a 19-year-old Caucasian male referred from his primary care physician for anxiety. Alec recently returned home after his first year of college. He reported that he did well academically but had issues with his roommate in his freshman year over a girl whom they both liked. He said that his roommate and several of his roommate's friends "jumped" him one evening. The attack resulted in Alec receiving 12 stiches on his forehead. University officials moved Alec to a new room. However, his former roommate was not suspended or expelled. His former roommate and his friends insisted that Alec started the fight. This seemed to shock Alec because he had expected to have a similar experience to that in high school where he was well-liked, played on the hockey team, and was the homecoming king. Alec will be transferring to another school for his sophomore year.

Alec had been in therapy before, when he was 12 years old, to manage his anxiety as he switched from a parochial to a public school. He and his mother (who was present for the initial session) said that after a few months of therapy and getting used to the new school, Alec did remarkably well. His former therapist used cognitive behavioral strategies to help Alec work through his anxiety, and Alec reports that he still uses these strategies today.

Alec's early development was typical, and his mother reports that he has always been a healthy kid. His parents are married and informed Alec that they will divorce within the year. Alec said that his parents have been living separate lives under the same roof (e.g., different bedrooms, separate vacations) for years now, and he is upset that they refuse to continue to live in this way. He seems devastated by the idea that his parents will divorce. Alec also has a younger brother, 11 years old, on the Autism Spectrum, and he worries what this will mean for his brother and his care.

Alec shared that he had been having frequent panic attacks where he feels like he cannot breathe, feels nauseous and/or dizzy, and has chest pain and heart palpitations. He had been to the local emergency department twice and insisted that he was having a heart attack. The emergency department sent Alec back to his primary care physician and then received a referral for therapy to work on his anxiety therapeutically. His primary care physician prescribed a trial of Xanax, which his mother administers when needed.

Alec works at a local trampoline park, where he has worked since his sophomore year of high school. Alec has many friends who work there too, and when Alec has a panic attack or severe anxiety, they often cover for him. Alec has recently feared driving because of the panic attacks and has been relying on his mother, father, and friends to drive him to work, therapy, and other places. He wants to quit working, but he is afraid to do so because he needs the money to pay for books and other incidentals in college. He feels that he needs to do this, particularly if his parents decide to divorce.

Alec recently started dating a girl who he had liked since high school. He was supposed to take her out and had planned an elaborate date. He never made it to the place that they were supposed to meet because he experienced a panic attack. When he called her later, she refused to speak to him. Since then, Alec has made repeated efforts to "win her back," but he has been unsuccessful.

■ DIAGNOSTIC IMPRESSIONS

Alec experienced a difficult first year in college and lived in fear of his roommate and others who physically assaulted him. His parents are also discussing the possibility of divorce, which will strain family finances and perhaps change his relationships with his parents. It seems that Alec, given his first-year exeperience, is fearful of his return to college at the end of the summer. He also seems embarrassed that he cannot stop the panic attacks and presents as angry with himself that he has to go through such lengths to control his mind.

■ DIAGNOSTIC CONCLUSIONS

Panic Disorder
Disruption of Family by Separation or Divorce

TREATMENT INTERVENTIONS

Psychopharmacology—Continue with medication management as prescribed with frequent monitoring from physician.
Therapy—Regular counseling sessions to help Alec monitor his symptoms and encourage him to develop coping skills to manage his anxiety.
Family therapy—Alec is struggling with his parents' impending divorce and what it means for their family. Working through his concerns with his family may be helpful to Alec and improve his symptoms.

■ UPDATE

Approximately 3 weeks into therapy, Alec mentioned that he has frequent neck pain. At this point, Alec had quit his job at the trampoline park because he felt guilty that his coworkers were doing his job, and Alec was getting "paid to panic in the employee lounge." When asked if he slept in an odd position as explanation of his neck pain, Alec said that he did a flip at the trampoline park when he first arrived home after freshman year. He said that he smacked his neck and head off the bar that supports the trampoline. Alec saw "stars" and then walked it off. It was recommended that Alec have an evaluation for head and neck injury. Alec was eventually diagnosed with a concussion.

■ DIAGNOSTIC CONCLUSIONS

Postconcussion Syndrome is a complex disorder in which various symptoms last for weeks and sometimes months after the injury that caused the concussion. It is not uncommon that brain injury results in headaches, dizziness, and other symptoms that mimic anxiety and panic disorders. As the brain recovers, symptoms subside. In Alec's case, they were nearly gone by the time he left to begin his sophomore year at a new university.

■ FOR YOUR CONSIDERATION

1. Part of the intake questionnaire asked if there had ever been any head or neck injuries. Alec reported that he had stitches after a fight during his freshman year of college, but no other injuries. How else would you find out about any potential head or medical injuries that may contribute to a client's current psychiatric symptoms?
2. Alec was relieved when he found out he "just" had a concussion. Why do you think that is? How does the differentiation of the body versus the mind contribute to stigma about mental health disorders?
3. Now that he has been diagnosed with a concussion, Alec and his parents think that discontinuation of therapy is best. Would you recommend that? Why or why not?

Billy

■ HISTORY

Billy is a 9-year-old Caucasian male who was brought to counseling by his mother, Tina. At the beginning of the session, Tina expressed concern regarding Billy's temper outburst and reluctance to follow rules. Tina mentioned that they moved to the area about 6 months ago owing to her husband's job relocating the family. They have adjusted well overall, but Billy has continued to be somewhat defiant and argumentative when redirected by his mother. Tina explained that her husband works a lot but that he is supportive of the consequences imposed by her when Billy does not listen. She also mentioned that Billy has been somewhat withdrawn and isolated since he started playing soccer with a local kids' team a month ago. Tina mentioned that the other children he was playing soccer with were not very nice and would pick on Billy. She worries that he is sad and is not sure how to help him.

During the interview, the counselor found out that Billy has been somewhat oppositional and defiant since the age of 3 years. He would argue with his parents, refuse to do what was asked of him, and then become really angry and throw things in his room. Billy blamed his parents for making him angry and for messing up his room. Although Billy does throw things in his room, he does not typically break things or damage his belongings or the house. Billy often also blamed his younger sister for annoying him. When Billy does become angry and explosive, it only lasts for up to 20 to 30 minutes and he usually calms down. He is not continuously upset, irritable, angry, or moody outside of the situations where he does not want to do what he is told. Interestingly, his mother indicated that Billy is an excellent student and behaves appropriately at school. Teachers praise Billy's behavioral compliance while in class. In addition, Tina stated that other parents also comment on Billy's behavior being so positive whenever he visits a friend or spends the night.

Billy took part in the interview without his mother present, which went well. He was respectful to the counselor and answered questions without hesitation. He willingly completed an age-appropriate depression scale (the Center for Epidemiological Studies Depression Scale for Children [CES-DC]) to explore the potential for depression given Tina's concerns about his mood. Tina completed the National Institute for Children's Health Quality (NICHQ) Vanderbilt Assessment Scale—Parent Informant to explore potential Attention-Deficit/Hyperactivity Disorder (ADHD) symptoms as well as some Disruptive Impulse-Control and Conduct Disorders (i.e., Oppositional Defiant Disorder [ODD] and Conduct Disorder). She also completed the *DSM-5* Emerging Measures Level 2—Parent/Guardian of Child Age 6 to 17 scales for both Depression and Anxiety (www.psychiatry.org/psychiatrists/practice/dsm/dsm-5/online-assessment-measures).

■ DIAGNOSTIC IMPRESSIONS

Considering the potential for different diagnoses or clinical struggles is important in the case of Billy. A thorough evaluation of Depressive Disorders, Disruptive Impulse-Control, and Conduct Disorders is warranted given that irritable mood may be present instead of a sad or depressed mood for children and adolescents struggling with Major Depressive Disorder (American Psychiatric Association [APA], 2013). Exploring Disruptive Mood Dysregulation Disorder is also important; however, Tina did clarify that Billy's mood is pleasant outside of the outbursts and does not persist as ". . . irritable or angry most of the day, nearly every day . . ." (APA, 2013, p. 156). Therefore, Criteria D for Disruptive Mood Dysregulation Disorder would not be met, and the diagnosis could be ruled out.

Tina mentioned that Billy's mood shifted to what she observes as sadness that started about a month ago when he started playing soccer. Exploring a Major Depressive Episode would be important, and Billy's CES-DC score was elevated (score of 19 [a cutoff of 15 indicating depressive symptoms]) and the Level 2—Parent/Guardian of Child Age 6 to 17 scale for Depression also indicated a Moderate level of depression (T-Score of 63.6). However, other than the sadness expressed by Billy's mother and Billy's own acknowledgment of feeling sad at times, Billy (and his mother) denied any complications with his eating, sleeping, energy level, lack of interest in activities, restlessness, or suicidal thoughts. They did, however, admit to some concentration struggles and feeling "less than" others (i.e., low self-esteem) to some degree. Three symptoms of Major Depressive Disorder are clearly identified in Billy's case—depressed or irritable mood, feeling more worthless than usual, and problems with concentration (APA, 2013, pp. 160–161). Still, the three symptoms are not enough to warrant a diagnosis of Major Depressive Disorder, for which five or more symptoms are required. A diagnosis of Adjustment Disorder with Depressed Mood would be appropriate given the three symptoms of depression, the depressive symptoms being exhibited after the experiences with his soccer team within 1 month of joining, the assessment results of the CES-DC and Level 2-Depression—Parent/Guardian of Child Age 6 to 17 scale, and the distress caused by the symptoms to the individual and the family system.

Billy's other area of concern surrounds the anger outburst and oppositional and defiant behaviors. Disruptive Mood Dysregulation Disorder has already been ruled out; however, other potential diagnoses need to be explored. An exploration of Disruptive Impulse-Control and Conduct Disorders provides some avenues to consider, including (A) ODD, (B) Conduct Disorder, and (C) Intermittent Explosive Disorder. The explanation of symptoms expressed by Tina and exhibited by Billy coincides with the diagnostic criteria for ODD. In order to be diagnosed with ODD, Billy must demonstrate at least four symptoms within the possible eight symptoms listed together with distress or impairment and the ruling out of other disorders (Bipolar Disorder, etc.; APA, 2013, p. 462). The case study clearly presents that Billy loses his temper, gets easily annoyed, becomes angry, argues with his parents (authority figures), refuses to follow

111

rules and directives, and blames others for his anger and misbe-haviors, which are all associated with the symptoms of ODD (APA, 2013, p. 462). Tina's concern and her own distress regarding Billy and his outbursts are clear indication of significant distress. In addition, Tina's completion of the NICHQ Vanderbilt Assessment Scale—Parent Informant provided some psychometric support for ODD, with five of the eight symptoms endorsed as occurring "Often" or "Very Often" as well as a "problematic" rating on the Relationship with Parents performance subscale. The results of the NICHQ Vanderbilt Assessment Scale—Parent Informant also indicated four symptoms of inattention and five symptoms of hyperactivity/impulsivity as endorsed with an "Often" or "Very Often" frequency; however, Billy's school behavior is always appropriate, and his academic functioning is exceptional. Therefore, the behaviors endorsed by Tina for Billy's NICHQ Vanderbilt Assessment Scale—Parent Informant are more associated with his oppositional behaviors. The *Diagnostic and Statistical Manual of Mental Disorders* (5th ed.; *DSM-5*; APA, 2013) cautions clinicians to be aware of this possibility in the differential diagnosis information for ADHD where it highlights how those diagnosed with ODD would refuse to follow the demands of authority figures but that symptom should be ". . . differentiated from aversion to school or mentally demanding tasks due to difficulty in sustaining mental effort, forgetting instructions, and impulsivity . . ." (APA, 2013, p. 63). Because Billy happily completes his homework and schoolwork while in class, he does not exhibit an aversion to work that requires mental effort. Because the symptoms of ODD are only present at home (one setting), the severity specifier would be Mild. Counselors will still want to rule out any other potential diagnosis prior to solidifying the ODD diagnosis.

Intermittent Explosive Disorder should be explored because of the arguments and temper tantrums (APA, 2013, p. 466). The frequency of verbal aggression would meet criteria A.1. (APA, 2013, p. 466), but the differential diagnosis information associated with Intermittent Explosive Disorder states "Aggression in oppositional defiant disorder is typically characterized by temper tantrums and verbal arguments with authority figures, whereas impulsive aggressive outbursts in intermittent explosive disorder are in response to a broader array of provocation and include physical assault" (APA, 2013, p. 469). Therefore, we can rule out Intermittent Explosive Disorder due to the verbal arguments occurring only with his parents and not within a variety of settings. In addition, Intermittent Explosive Disorder requires that the outbursts are not focused on getting something (criteria C; APA, 2013, p. 466), but Billy usually has his temper tantrums and outbursts when he does not want to do something and is trying to intimidate his mother into giving up and allowing him not to follow the directive. Lastly, Conduct Disorder is explored; however, the symptoms and criteria for Conduct Disorder are much more severe than what Billy is exhibiting. Therefore, Conduct Disorder can be easily ruled out.

■ DIAGNOSTIC CONCLUSIONS

Oppositional Defiant Disorder, Mild
Adjustment Disorder With Depressed Mood

■ SUGGESTED THERAPEUTIC INTERVENTIONS

Counselors are encouraged to consider the culture of the child and/or family system when working with individuals diagnosed with ODD. Cultural considerations will help clinicians better determine the most appropriate intervention. Some interventions that have proved to be beneficial in general include cognitive behavioral therapy (CBT) (Battagliese et al., 2015) and behavioral interventions via parent education and training (Kledzik, Thorne, Prasad, Hayes, & Hines, 2012). CBT may be helpful in providing a combination of efforts focused on changing the thought processes of the client and/or the family system. Battagliese et al. (2015) conducted a meta-analysis of 21 studies that explored either a cognitive behavioral, cognitive, or behavioral intervention. The authors combined all three approaches and cohesively identified them as CBT. The CBT interventions within the 21 studies were specifically focused on externalizing behaviors that included ADHD, ODD, and Conduct Disorder. The meta-analysis included 10 factors such as ODD symptoms, parental stress, and aggressive behaviors (Battagliese et al., 2015). Results of the meta-analysis did provide support for the use of CBT interventions for reduction of

ODD symptoms based on parent report measures (Battagliese et al., 2015). However, CBT may be difficult to implement depending on the age of the client diagnosed with ODD and/or the client's openness to exploring his or her own role in the struggle. Therefore, behavioral interventions are also considered and often touted as the initial treatment approach when it comes to addressing ODD (Kledzik et al., 2012).

Some concepts presented by Kledzik et al. (2012) included how verbal praise and other forms of positive reinforcements tend to help parents and children change their negative interaction cycle to healthier dynamics (p. 559). Included in the behavioral interventions are parent trainings to help them better approach their child with rules and rewards. The authors recommended prioritizing behaviors (2 or 3) and to phrase the rules for behaviors in "do" versus "don't" terminology (Kledzik et al., 2012, p. 559). For example, instead of saying, "don't touch anything that doesn't belong to you," say, "only touch things that belong to you." Lastly, Kledzik et al. (2012) explained that regular information on psychopharmacological interventions for children solely diagnosed with ODD was not available but that those who have comorbid ADHD often do benefit from stimulant medication and/or atomoxetine for impulse control.

In Billy's case, his parents would be provided with behavior modification training focused on implementing rules with specific consequences. They would be encouraged to use choice terminology that would emphasize the personal responsibility of Billy in his experience of consequences (Dean, 2015). An example of choice terminology focused on emphasizing the positive reinforcement is "Billy, if you choose to put up your clean clothes within the next 10 minutes, you choose to watch television for an hour today." An example of how the choice terminology emphasizes the personal responsibility is "Billy, you did not choose to put up your clean clothes within the 10 minutes allotted; therefore, you chose to give up 15 minutes of your television time." Parents would be encouraged to fragment positive reinforcements and avoid all-or-nothing consequences to allow the child (Billy) to still see that he has something he can work toward if he would choose to follow the rules. Billy's parents would be provided with detailed guidelines; however, they would be encouraged to adjust the behavior modification plan to fit their family personality as well as the components that work best with Billy.

■ FOR YOUR CONSIDERATION

Billy's parents would be asked to continue to monitor his symptoms of depression and ODD. Counselors can continue to explore whether depressive and/or ODD symptoms are still present through both clinical interviews and/or readministration of the assessment measures completed during the initial visit.

1. If Billy and his family were African American or Hispanic, would you have any diagnostic considerations based on possible cultural factors?
2. If Billy's depressive symptoms increased or grew more severe, would you change any of his diagnoses? If so, what disorder(s) come to mind?
3. If Billy's disruptive behaviors became more severe to include stealing and sneaking out at night, would you change or add any diagnoses? If so, what would you consider?

■ REFERENCES

American Psychiatric Association. (2013). *Diagnostic and statistical manual of mental disorders* (5th ed.). Arlington, VA: American Psychiatric Publishing.

Battagliese, G., Caccetta, M., Luppino, O. I., Baglioni, C., Cardi, V., Mancini, F., & Buonanno, C. (2015). Cognitive-behavioral therapy for externalizing disorders. *Behavior Research and Therapy, 75*, 60–71.

Dean, C. J. (2015, February). *Addressing problematic behaviors in children: Integrating behavioral family therapy & choice theory.* Presented at the Louisiana Association for Marriage and Family Therapy Annual Conference, Baton Rouge, Louisiana.

Kledzik, A. M., Thorne, M. C., Prasad, V., Hayes, K. H., & Hines, L. (2012). Challenges in treating oppositional defiant disorder in a pediatric medical setting: A case study. *Journal of Pediatric Nursing, 27*, 557–562. doi:10.1016/j.pedn.2011.06.006

Jack

■ HISTORY

Jack is a 45-year-old, married father of two grown-up children and two stepchildren. Jack is a real estate entrepreneur who is co-owner of a real estate brokerage firm. Jack is married to his second wife, Suzanne, who is a respected professor at a major university in their community. Suzanne discovered Jack was having an affair when she logged on to his computer while hers was being repaired. A week after discovering the affair, the bank notified Suzanne of a large overdraft on their joint investment account. Until the discovery of the affair, Suzanne thought they had "the perfect marriage."

Jack indicates he had come to counseling to "save my marriage." He reports Suzanne is devastated and is seeking individual counseling to cope with the betrayal. Jack says he has not been able to sleep since Suzanne found out about the affair and swears that woman "meant nothing to me. It was just a time when I was so distracted about the biggest deal I have ever worked, and she was, frankly, flirting with me for quite a while. She is new in the business and asked for my advice. One thing led to another—that stuff happens—but I don't want to end our marriage."

When asked about the overdraft, Jack says he was just a little short of funding, and it is no big deal. He insists he will pay it back. "That is just part of this business." Jack reports he is a successful real estate broker who has been ranked in the top 10 producers in his community for the past 5 years. He prides himself on being one of the best in his business and hopes his adult son will join the firm. "You gotta be willing to take risks. Not everyone is willing to do what it takes, and that's why I've been tops in this business. When this deal closes I'll be number 1 and be honored at our yearly banquet."

His business partner is a woman who, as Jack reports, "was at first a real friend and we did all our deals together, but she began to question me on how I put our deals together, and now we rarely speak to each other." He hopes she will leave the firm but sees no room for negotiation at this time. "I just close my door and don't speak to her unless it is absolutely necessary. She'll be sorry when she falls flat on her face without me helping her create the deals."

Jack reported he has always had a tremendous amount of energy. "As a kid I was always in some sort of trouble for having too much fun." Jack reports he was arrested at the age of 15 for underage drinking and racing his four–wheeler along a creek in a residential neighborhood. He reportedly did community service, and the incident was erased from his record when he turned 18 years old. "I was bored in high school and by my senior year, I was skipping as often as I could. I never got caught and the teachers would get furious because I still made good grades on my tests. I think I was more intelligent than most of them and they knew it. We used to go to Mr. Ted's grocery and steal a couple of beers and head to the pool. He never figured us out, but when I was old enough to buy beer legally, I would stop by and buy beer or get some milk. I figured that made us even."

Jack currently plays competitive tennis and lifts weights at a local gym. He reports drinking occasionally but alleges no drug use. He does receive testosterone injections "to keep my energy up." Jack concluded by stating, "I'll do whatever you tell me to do. I don't want another divorce."

After obtaining permission to speak to Jack's wife, Suzanne, she revealed that she often worried about Jack's financial dealings and knew he often "rolled the dice" but was confident he would never put their personal finances at risk. Now she is not so sure. She says she was attracted to Jack for his personality. "He was always the life of the party and never met a stranger. He was ambitious and knew how to get things done. I knew he would be a success. I never dreamed he would cheat on me."

She further revealed Jack had a previous bankruptcy and re-organization of his company, which resulted in a long-term lawsuit with his former partner. She added, "He's not like that at home. He always remembers my birthday and our anniversary and buys me wonderful gifts. Last year he gave me and my daughters a trip to Las Vegas. He was always so generous with them—they adore him." Suzanne shared that Jack is not close to his youngest son because he sided with his mother in their divorce. His first wife is reportedly still bitter about Jack leaving the family.

■ DIAGNOSTIC IMPRESSIONS

There is often a fine line between irresponsibility and criminal activity. Most of us have participated in some illegal behavior at one time or another, but with little harm to others and few consequences. Who has not gone above the posted speed limit or cruised through a stop sign when no cars were in sight? However, one can begin to place patterns of behavior on a spectrum of irresponsibility. Some behaviors are irresponsible and out of the cultural norms but are not criminal and thus are *nonarrestable*. Further across the spectrum are the *arrestable* behaviors ranging from white-collar crime to violent acts of aggression.

Jack, like most psychopaths, has a long history of irresponsible and sometimes criminal behavior, which pervades his life and has caused distress to those around him. Jack clearly demonstrates this pattern of irresponsibility, beginning in his adolescent years with high-risk behaviors and a disregard for rules and regulations. Yet he prides himself on being a good person in spite of his questionable business practices and his recently revealed infidelity. He has a history of conflicted relationships and is quick to blame others for the conflict. Jack appears to be concerned about his image in maintaining the marriage with little empathy for Suzanne's distress. Jack relishes the adoration of his stepdaughters and emphasizes his success by buying expensive gifts and trips, although he rarely spends time with any of his family.

■ DIAGNOSTIC CONCLUSIONS

Although the person with an Antisocial Personality Disorder may have many of the features of a Narcissistic Personality Disorder, the distinguishing features for a diagnosis of Antisocial Personality Disorder are irritability or aggressiveness, deceitfulness, lying, and irresponsible or unlawful behavior throughout his or her history. Another distinction may be made between a person who is educated with a viable career and who takes calculated risks, and another who is disenfranchised, lacks opportunity and education, and commits impulsive criminal acts out of rage toward an oppressive environment. Although neither is excused from responsibility, there is an environmental factor to be acknowledged with the latter.

The *DSM-5* diagnosis may be the same for each, but the treatment options are markedly different. One client will likely obtain legal counsel and be seen in a private practice or chic counseling setting, whereas the latter will find themselves using whatever mental health and legal services are available in the criminal justice system.

> Antisocial Personality Disorder
> Other Problems Related to Employment

■ SUGGESTED THERAPEUTIC INTERVENTIONS

Traditional empathic counseling strategies are ineffective with this population. The counselor must have a working knowledge of the thought processes of the psychopath for any chance of creating an opportunity for change. The thinking is continuous, and fantasies of power and control are pervasive. Jack likely has many more irresponsible behaviors, which he does not intend to reveal. He probably does not want a divorce, either because he does not want to share his wealth or he wants to maintain his image. The psychopath keeps attachments as long as the relationship is to his or her advantage (including with the counselor).

The counselor must investigate the underlying reason for counseling through deductive reasoning. One should assume Jack's goal is not to change but to pacify others for some hidden agenda. The only time that change is possible is when the psychopath is vulnerable.

This opportunity may come for Jack if further business failures, legal implications, or loss of his wealth and/or image is at risk.

Underlying the grandiosity is extreme fear, which is kept at bay at all costs. There appears to be such an inner void that some have termed the dreaded state a *zero* state. However, the counseling strategy should be primarily focused on Jack's thinking and the ultimate responsibility for his behavior. The goal is to create transparency into Jack's thought processes. As the consequences of the irresponsible behavior are pointed out to the client, a typical response is "Everyone does it." The counselor must find a balance between confronting each "con" and remaining nonjudgmental. The first "con" in Jack's presentation is "Tell me what to do."

■ FOR YOUR CONSIDERATION

1. Could Jack become suicidal when and if he becomes vulnerable to his inner fears? Would hospitalization be beneficial?
2. Would having access to significant others in Jack's life be beneficial to know the extent of Jack's irresponsibility? How might this affect the counseling?
3. How will Jack con you? After all, counselors are good at establishing trust through rapport, aren't we? Good counseling is all about the therapeutic relationship. Or is it?

Luz

■ HISTORY

Luz is a 43-year-old female born in Nicaragua who became an American citizen after studying physical therapy in the United States. She has been living in the United States for 26 years and is married to a U.S. Federal Marshall who is a 58-year-old Caucasian male. Her religious faith is Roman Catholic, and she explained that her faith is a strong component of her life. She came to counseling owing to sexual problems in her marriage and wants to be "happy with her husband again." Her husband, David, had a previous marriage from which he has two children who are now adults. David and Luz have one child together, a 10-year-old daughter named Elizabeth, who lives with them. During her pregnancy with Elizabeth, David's other children came to live with them, which caused some transitional stresses. Some of the challenges with the transition were the result of David's ex-wife making negative statements about Luz to the children who avoided her and rejected her attempts at developing a relationship. In addition, Luz had a very difficult and complicated pregnancy and childbirth.

Upon the delivery of Elizabeth, David took notice of Luz's struggles and informed her that he would not put her in such a predicament again. However, when Luz heard this, she interpreted the message as a negative statement. Thereafter, as she reflected on what David said, she thought to herself: "I'll make sure it never happens again." Since that moment of reflection, Luz and David have not had sexual intercourse or any other sexually oriented touching, though they are physically affectionate, with limitations, and do hold hands. They are respectful to each other, but whenever David tries to cuddle with her, Luz quickly turns away owing to fears that he may try to turn the cuddling into a sexual advance.

David joined Luz for a couples' session since the struggle presented as a systemic concern. David would like to retire and move to another state but is insistent on a full emotional, physical, and spiritual relationship together before he commits to them moving as a family. David has been patient for the past 10 years but is increasingly becoming frustrated with the lack of her willingness to engage in physical intimacy. Luz stated that she has a low libido, and after a physical exam from her gynecologist, there were no physical reasons for her libido to be low. The gynecologist ruled out early menopause or any other physical conditions that would contribute to a low libido and suggested counseling to explore any mental health barriers.

■ DIAGNOSTIC IMPRESSIONS

Simons and Carey (2001) conducted an extensive literature review of 10 years of data on the prevalence of sexual dysfunctions for both men and women. Two studies within their literature review are pertinent to the prevalence of Female Sexual Arousal Disorder for women in the United States. Laumann, Paik, and Rosen (1999) reported a 1-year study of prevalence of Female Sexual Arousal Disorder that indicated 19% in a representative U.S. sample. However, Chandraiah, Levenson, and Collins (1991) reported a lifetime prevalence of 21% in a primary care setting based on *DSM-III* criteria.

Female sexual dysfunction in general is a complex and little understood condition affecting women of all ages and ethnicities. According to Markovic (2010), several factors may influence sexual desire, including "life experiences, stresses and anxiety; body image; communication issues; economic situation; sexual education; belief system, sexual technique and habits; cultural expectations." (p. 260). Comorbidity may present as Mood and/or Anxiety disorders, panic attacks, depression, phobias, or bipolar disorder (Hurlbert et al., 2005).

Women with low sexual desire often have low self-image and mood instability (Basson, Brotto, Laan, Redmond, & Utian, 2005). Specific knowledge of these factors is pertinent for the clinician in developing a treatment plan for the disorder, with a goal of improvement in the enjoyment of sexual activity by the client. As illustrated by the case of Luz, what may be often overlooked is the role that a closeted memory can play in inhibiting sexual enjoyment and thus precipitating individual stressors as well as marital discord.

During the diagnostic process, Luz admitted to never really having much interest in sex. She recalls as a young woman how her coworkers would discuss their sexual escapades and how she did not find such experiences interesting or exciting. Luz admitted to being willing to engage in sexual physical contact with David upon their marriage but explained that she wanted to be a mother, which was the motivating factor for her willingness to be sexual with David. Still, she never initiated physical intimacy. She denied ever having had any sexual fantasies regarding anybody, and unfortunately not even her husband. She does feel a little guilty that she has not desired her husband physically, although she does love him and adores him in many other ways. Luz explains that sexual intercourse was neither pleasant nor painful, but it was uncomfortable to some degree owing to feeling inadequate for not feeling pleasure. She also feels guilty for avoiding sexual contact with David because of the lack of pleasure and discomfort she felt during sex. Luz feels as though she cannot win because she feels guilty either way, but she worries more about David thinking he cannot satisfy her during intercourse and the potential resulting impact on his self-esteem. Therefore, she prefers to avoid sexual contact and work through the guilt by loving David in other ways (caretaker, homemaker, etc.), which she gladly takes on in addition to her work. Luz highlighted that she would love to be able to enjoy sex and for it to not be so unfulfilling and uncomfortable but does not know exactly how to make that happen. When questioned about her attempts to address the problem, she explains that she has avoided working on it with David because of her past experiences and inability to enjoy sex or feel aroused and the subsequent guilt she experieced when sex was over.

Luz completed the Female Sexual Distress Scale—Revised (FSDS-R) resulting with a total score of 27 (a score of 11 and above helps differentiate between Female Sexual Dysfunction [FSD] and no FSD). In addition, exploring the diagnostic criteria for Female Sexual Interest/Arousal Disorder provides a clear indication that Luz meets several of the criteria to include a lack of interest (or reduced interest) in sexual activities, lack of sexual thoughts and fantasies, lack of initiation in sexual activity, and being unreceptive to sexual advances from her husband (American Psychiatric Association [APA], 2013). However, in order to ensure an accurate diagnosis, a differential diagnostic process was applied.

Given the lack of sexual desire that can be present with other mental disorders, such as Major Depression, Luz was questioned regarding her overall mood presentation. She denied feeling sad or having other symptoms of depression such as fatigue, difficulty concentrating, or lack of interest in activities (APA, 2013) with the exception of feeling guilty about her lack of sexual involvement with her husband. She completed the *DSM-5* Emerging Measures Level 2—Adult form, for Depression (www.psychiatry.org/psychiatrists/practice/dsm/dsm-5/online-assessment-measures) with an overall score of 12, indicating no significant level of depression. The items that she endorsed as "sometimes" were associated with feeling sad and hopeless. When questioned about her answers, Luz explained that it usually occurred after David approached her for sexual intimacy and she would decline his advancement. She further clarified that such feelings were often associated with her guilt and feeling hopeless about the possibility of a sexually satisfying relationship for her marriage.

Luz was also questioned about possible avoidance associated with trauma reactions and Posttraumatic Stress Disorder (APA, 2013). However, Luz denied feeling as though her life or the life of the child was ever in real danger during the pregnancy or delivery. She said that she has not had any unpleasant dreams about the pregnancy or childbirth and that she is fine talking about the experience because it resulted with a very positive outcome—the birth of her child. Luz did not demonstrate any other symptoms associated with any other mental disorder. Luz does drink on occasions, but her drinking is so infrequent and without any related symptoms associated with any Substance Use Disorders. In addition, since her doctor completed a panel of tests and a thorough examination regarding her physical health, medical conditions were also ruled out.

Given Luz's cultural background, the concept of *marianismo* was explored. Sanchez, Whittaker, Hamilton, and Zayas (2016) defined *marianismo* as "a gender role construct that describes the expectations and norms for some Latina women (and girls) based on a collectivistic worldview in which interdependence and familial hierarchy are the cultural norm" (p. 396). The authors further explained that the potential negative component of *marianismo* "may reinforce sexual silence and the avoidance of communication about sexually intimate behaviors" (Sanchez et al., 2016, p. 397). Although the Sanchez et al. (2016) study was mainly focused on adolescent girls hypothesizing that such negative components would contribute to sexual engagement in order to reduce distress in romantic relationships, the concept of avoidance was specifically applied to Luz because she was not willing to engage in sexual intimacy with David beyond the birth of their first child together. Luz admitted to her strong religious beliefs as a factor when she was a younger girl but denied any contributions of *marianismo* factors to her lack of sexual interest or arousal.

■ DIAGNOSTIC CONCLUSIONS

Female Sexual Interest/Arousal Disorder, Lifelong, Generalized, Moderate

■ SUGGESTED THERAPEUTIC INTERVENTIONS

Treating Female Sexual Interest/Arousal Disorder is complicated by the fact that there is rarely a single causative factor that can be traced as the reason for the problem, and this is exacerbated by the fact that there are limited psychotherapy treatment options. A review of published articles highlights the plethora of studies associated with addressing abnormal physiological findings. A review of the literature gleans some studies of recommended psychotherapy approaches with encouraging outcomes.

Treatment of clients who meet the *DSM-5* criteria for Female Sexual Interest/Arousal Disorder requires an individualized approach that may include a combination of counseling, cognitive behavioral interventions, pharmacotherapy, and/or remedies for concomitant medical or psychiatric conditions (Graham, 2010). Pharmacological treatments such as hormone therapy may be options for treating physiological needs, imbalances, or other symptomatic complaints, and comprise one part of the overall treatment management of clients with female sexual disorders.

The family doctor will likely refer a client to a qualified specialist, who may be a sex therapist or a psychotherapist specializing in behavior modification or cognitive behavior therapy. As the case of Luz represents, some clients state that their reason for seeking treatment is that if they could increase their own level of desire, it would be easier to deal with their partner's sexual demands. "The key for successful therapy evidently lies in identifying the 'motivations (reasons/incentives)' for being willing to attempt to become sexually aroused by their partners in order to experience responsive sexual desire and then enhancing those motivations" (Basson et al., 2005, as cited in Durr, 2009, p. 299).

Therapy may include education about how to optimize the body's sexual response, ways to enhance intimacy with their partner, and recommendations for reading materials or couples' exercises (Palacios, Castano, & Grazziotin, 2009). Cognitive behavioral therapy and sensate focus techniques (progression from nonsexual contact up to sexual touching, similar to systematic desensitization but focused on resensitizing) are useful therapies (Basson et al., 2005). A mindfulness program designed by Brotto and Barker (2014) incorporates Buddhist principles to establish a connection between the mind and body. The program includes education in the basics of mindfulness meditation, practicing mindfulness for a period of time, along with the woman engaging in observation and examination of her body in nonsexual ways. In addition, engagement in reducing distracting thoughts, that is, judgments about their physical appearance, is another component of the program. The mindfulness program has been shown to be successful by women with various sexual disorders.

■ FOR YOUR CONSIDERATION

1. Would you consider Luz's condition a disorder? Do you believe that diagnoses like Female Sexual Interest/Arousal Disorder should be included in the *DSM-5*?
2. What other diagnoses, if any, would you consider for Luz if she were from a different culture? Why?
3. If Luz were unresponsive to recommended treatment, would you change any aspect of her diagnosis? If so, what diagnoses come to mind?

■ REFERENCES

American Psychiatric Association. (2013). *Diagnostic and statistical manual of mental disorders* (5th ed.). Arlington, VA: American Psychiatric Publishing.

Basson, R., Brotto, L. A., Laan, E., Redmond, G., & Utian, W. H. (2005). Assessment and management of women's sexual dysfunctions: Problematic desire and arousal. *Journal of Sexual Medicine, 2,* 291–300.

Brotto, L. A., & Barker, M., (Eds.). (2014). *Mindfulness in sexual and relationship therapy.* Abingdon, United Kingdom: Routledge.

Chandraiah, S., Levenson, J. L., & Collins, J. B. (1991). Sexual dysfunction, social maladjustment, and psychiatric disorders in women seeking treatment in a premenstrual syndrome clinic. *International Journal of Psychiatry in Medicine, 21,* 189–204.

Durr, E. (2009). Lack of 'responsive' sexual desire in women: Implications for clinical practice. *Sexual and Relationship Therapy, 24*(3–4), 292–306.

Graham, C. (2010). The *DSM* diagnostic criteria for female sexual arousal disorder. *Archives of Sexual Behavior, 39*(2), 240–255.

Hurlbert, D. F., Fertel, E. R., Singh, D., Fernandez, F., Menendez, D., & Salgado, C. (2005). The role of sexual functioning in the sexual desire adjustment and psychosocial adaptation of women with hypoactive sexual desire. *The Canadian Journal of Human Sexuality, 14*(1–2), 15–30.

Laumann, E. O., Paik, A., & Rosen, R. C. (1999). Sexual dysfunction in the United States. *The Journal of the American Medical Association, 281,* 537–544.

Markovic, D. (2010). Hypoactive sexual desire disorder: Can it be treated by drugs? *Sexual and Relationship Therapy, 25*(3), 259–263.

Palacios, S., Castano, R., & Grazziotin, A. (2009). Epidemiology of female sexual dysfunction. *Maturitas, 63*(2), 119–123.

Sanchez, D., Whittaker, T. A., Hamilton, E., & Zayas, L. H. (2016). Perceived discrimination and sexual precursor behaviors in Mexican American preadolescent girls: The role of psychological distress, sexual attitudes, and marianismo beliefs. *Cultural Diversity and Ethnic Minority Psychology, 22*(3), 395-407. doi:10.1037/cdp0000066

Simons, J., & Carey, M. P. (2001). Prevalence of sexual dysfunctions: Results from a decade of research. *Archives of Sexual Behavior, 30*(2), 177–219.

Nathan

■ HISTORY

Nathan, a 17-year-old male high school student, has isolated himself from other males and spends the majority of his socializing with female friends. Nathan goes out of his way to avoid being alone with other males, including teachers and coworkers at his part-time job. He recently quit the men's basketball team because it required him to be in such close contact with other males.

Nathan identifies as heterosexual, yet he constantly worries that he might be gay. He runs through scenarios that would provide him an opportunity for physical or sexual contact with other males and then checks in with himself to determine whether or not he would find that contact pleasurable, or more pleasurable than what he would have with a female. He has watched gay pornography online to determine whether or not he would be turned on or achieve orgasm. Because he does not orgasm, he views this as confirmation that he is straight.

He harbors some guilt for rejecting his male friends, and his former best friend in particular, who has asked Nathan why he does not call him or want to hang out anymore. The friend wondered what he did wrong, and Nathan, not knowing what to say, said nothing to him. Nathan mentioned that when he sees his former teammates walking together in the hallways, he feels wistful, but then he quickly justifies why it "had to be done."

An only child of two progressive parents, Nathan shared his anguish with them. They asked him if he were gay and told him that if he were gay, that would be fine with them. Nathan was distressed by their reaction and took their open stance as, "My parents think I am gay."

Nathan is obsessive about how he conveys himself to others at his affluent, suburban high school. He wears clothing that purposely conveys a "straight" persona and aims to speak in a manner that demonstrates a flat affect. He is a skilled writer but does not think he should participate in the student literary magazine because "that would be gay." He is constantly assessing what he does, thinks, wears, and feels against whether or not that means he is gay or straight.

Nathan requested counseling services for himself to work through his concern about his sexuality. His parents, wishing for him to be healthy no matter what, complied with his request.

■ DIAGNOSTIC IMPRESSIONS

Nathan seems to be suffering from Sexual Orientation Obsession, a manifestation of Obsessive Compulsive Disorder (OCD) that revolves around the fear of being or being perceived as gay. This is different from Internalized Homophobia, in which someone who is actually lesbian, gay, or bisexual suffers personal and social anxiety over his or her sexual orientation. In this case, by contrast, Nathan does not take pleasure in homosexual thoughts but nonetheless has an obsessive need to reassure himself that he does not find them pleasurable.

OCD is characterized by the presence of obsessions and/or compulsions. Obsessions are recurrent and persistent thoughts (e.g., Am I gay?) that are experienced as intrusive and unwanted. Compulsions are repetitive behaviors (e.g., checking appearance for "straightness," watching gay pornography to assess reaction) that an individual feels driven to perform in response to an obsession or according to rules that must be applied rigidly.

■ DIAGNOSTIC CONCLUSION

Obsessive Compulsive Disorder

■ SUGGESTED THERAPEUTIC INTERVENTIONS

Psychopharmacology—Selective serotonin reuptake inhibitors to improve mood and assist Nathan in working through issues therapeutically.

Outpatient Therapy—Cognitive behavioral therapy to help Nathan change faulty ideas and beliefs, including those prevalent in this form of OCD.

■ FOR YOUR CONSIDERATION

1. How would you be able to tell the difference between Nathan's manifestation of OCD versus. Internalized Homophobia?
2. How would you counsel Nathan's parents if they participated in a family session with Nathan? Do you think their initial response was helpful or hurtful to Nathan? Explain.

Bryant

■ HISTORY

Bryant, a 20-year-old male college student, sought treatment for his voyeuristic urges after he was caught by his roommate "peering" across the quad at the girls' dormitory with binoculars. The roommate threatened to report him, and Bryant is concerned that he will lose his college scholarship and be expelled from the university.

Bryant articulated that he has no problems attracting sexual partners and has an active sex life. He reports that he hooks up, on average, one or two times per week. However, these sexual relationships do not provide Bryant with the level of pleasure that he gains from his voyeuristic endeavors. He reports that he began voyeurism in junior high school when he had a new neighbor move in and he could see her bedroom from his bedroom window. The neighbor, a young woman, did not shut her blinds, and Bryant viewed this as an invitation to watch her change clothing, apply beauty products, and have sex.

With the binoculars and, at times, night-vision goggles, Bryant admitted peering into the windows of the dormitories on campus, local apartments, and sorority houses to watch females undressing or having sex. When Bryant finds a suitable target, he masturbates to orgasm either while he watches or shortly thereafter. Bryant has not pursued sexual relationships with the women he observes and denies that this is his goal. He denies any plans, impulses, or fantasies to engage in rape. Bryant endorses pleasure from the voyeuristic act, and the threat of being caught makes it "hotter" for him.

On several occasions, Bryant was nearly caught by a bystander or one of his targets. He was shocked that his roommate caught him in the act and blames his target for "taking so long" as the reason for his roommate walking in on him. Bryant feels neither guilty nor ashamed about his voyeuristic tendencies and says that he is not harming anyone. However, given the current legal landscape toward sexual offenders, Bryant is motivated to seek help to change his sexual behavior.

■ DIAGNOSTIC IMPRESSIONS

Bryant's desire to watch others in sexual situations is common; there is an entire industry—pornography—built around the idea that people like to watch others having sex. Voyeurism usually begins during adolescence or early adulthood. In Bryant's case, his voyeurism is pathological, and he spends a considerable amount of time seeking out viewing opportunities to the exclusion of other important responsibilities and relationships. It seems that Bryant's voyeurism developed accidentally and now seems to be a method of achieving orgasm.

Voyeuristic Disorder is a *paraphilic disorder*—disorders that cause distress or impairment to the individual or entail a risk of personal harm. In the *Diagnostic and Statistical Manual of Mental Disorders* (5th ed.; *DSM-5;* American Psychiatric Association, 2013) it is said that up to 12% of males and 4% of females may meet clinical criteria for Voyeuristic Disorder; most do not seek medical evaluation and treatment unless compelled.

■ DIAGNOSTIC CONCLUSIONS

Voyeuristic Disorder
Potential problems with university authorities, legal system; tension in living situation

■ SUGGESTED THERAPEUTIC INTERVENTIONS

Psychopharmacology to diminish these unusual sexual urges.

Behavioral Therapy to encourage those with impulse control difficulties to control their urge to watch nonconsenting targets.

Social Skills Training to acquire more acceptable and harmless ways of sexual gratification.

■ FOR YOUR CONSIDERATION

1. Would you consider an individual like Bryant to be a sexual predator? Why or why not?
2. Is pornography simply a legalized version of voyeurism? Why or why not?

Adrienne

■ HISTORY

Adrienne is a 14-year-old Caucasian female of Greek descent. She is the youngest of three children and is in the eighth grade in a large, suburban middle school. Her mother brought her into the initial session after a referral from Adrienne's dermatologist, who had been treating her cystic acne for over a year. The dermatologist was concerned that Adrienne was scratching and picking at her cysts, and thus, they were not healing properly.

Adrienne presented with pigmentation and large cysts over her face, neck, and chest. She noted that she has an intense urge to pick at and scratch her face during times of stress at school and said she was often relieved after the cyst popped and her skin bled.

When Adrienne was 5 years old, her mother and older brothers left her father and stayed with her maternal grandparents, with whom they still reside. Adrienne's father was physically and verbally abusive to her mother and brothers, although not to Adrienne, per self-report. Adrienne said that even though she knew that her father was "not always nice" to the other members of the family, he was kind to her and she missed him when they left the home. She said that she used to have visits with him, but those tapered off after the divorce was finalized.

Approximately 2 years ago, when she was 12 years old, Adrienne learned from a family friend that her father had remarried and had two daughters with his new wife. This family friend showed Adrienne a smiling family photo from social media of her father with his wife and two small daughters. Adrienne said that she felt a lot of emotions in that moment, but the biggest one was that she was worthless.

Adrienne had "always" picked her skin, per self-report and that of her mother who said that she worried anytime Adrienne had a scratch or mosquito bite—her picking at the lesion would make it 10 times worse. However, after learning of the news about her father, the picking worsened, and Adrienne began picking at small pimples, whiteheads, and blackheads on her skin. She reportedly "pops" the hairs out of her eyebrows and in between her eyebrows too.

In terms of peer relationships, Adrienne has a handful of friends and plays softball for the school team. She is the catcher for the team and said that her coach probably allowed her to be the catcher because the "catcher's mask covers" her face. She is teased by many of the kids in her school and painfully recalled how a small child once asked her how she "got marbles stuck in her face."

When asked if she wants treatment to manage the urge to pick, Adrienne was ambivalent. She does not want to look the way that she does, as evidenced by her visits to the dermatologist and using prescription acne medication. On the other hand, she reports pleasurable feelings from picking her skin and feels a release when she is able to pick successfully (e.g., pop a zit, remove a blackhead).

■ DIAGNOSTIC IMPRESSIONS

Adrienne presents as moderately anxious. She admits to a low frustration tolerance and snaps at others over small matters, such as when others are 5 minutes late to a meeting. Her mother reports that she is often irritable for "no reason," but when she picks she seems to calm down. She also has difficulty sleeping even though she is easily fatigued. Thus, Adrienne seems to endorse excoriation as a way to cope with intense emotional distress.

The specific *DSM-5* criteria for Excoriation (Skin-Picking) Disorder are as follows:

- Recurrent skin picking resulting in lesions
- Repeated attempts to decrease or stop skin picking

- The skin picking causes clinically significant distress or impairment in important areas of functioning
- The skin picking cannot be attributed to the physiological effects of a substance or another medical condition
- The skin picking cannot be better explained by the symptoms of another mental disorder

Adrienne seems to meet the aforementioned criteria and does not meet criteria for Obsessive Compulsive Disorder. Thus, Excoriation Disorder is the appropriate diagnosis; rule out Generalized Anxiety Disorder.

■ DIAGNOSTIC CONCLUSIONS

Excoriation (Skin-Picking) Disorder
R/O Generalized Anxiety Disorder
Lack of coping skills, difficulty with peer relationships, and estrangement from father

■ SUGGESTED THERAPEUTIC INTERVENTIONS

Behavioral Techniques such as habit reversal, distraction, and mindfulness may mitigate the skin picking urge.

Psychopharmacology, such as a selective serotonin reuptake inhibitor, may provide assistance in managing the urge to pick and feelings of inadequacy.

■ FOR YOUR CONSIDERATION

1. Adrienne's skin picking worsened when she learned that her father had a new family. Why do you think, after all this time, Adrienne would be so triggered by this information?
2. In Adrienne's case, Excoriation Disorder was diagnosed with cystic acne and topical acne medication was pescribed over a year before the referral to a mental health professional. Why do you think it took so long to get Adrienne the treatment that she needed?

Jacob

■ HISTORY

Jacob is a 9-year-old male who lives with his mother, father, and two sisters aged 15 and 17 years. Jacob's mother presented for the initial intake session without Jacob to discuss concerns she had regarding Jacob and to determine whether counseling would be beneficial. Jacob is in the third grade at a public elementary school in a suburban setting. Jacob's mother, Patricia, reported that Jacob struggles in the home setting as well as in school—both academically and with peers.

Patricia reported that from the time he was a toddler, Jacob has been "different from the other kids." Although Jacob started speaking around the age of 2 years, Patricia reports that he used his words mainly to get what he wanted and he did not seem to be interested in talking for any other reason. Patricia reports that he did not use his words to express thoughts or feelings like her other children. He would often get upset (tantruming) over minor things—not having a particular cup or changing brands of common items. Jacob never asked "why" questions or appeared interested in engaging with others unless he needed or wanted something. Patricia notes that Jacob was often the child who played alone at birthday parties or family get-togethers. Jacob often resisted interacting with the other kids or failed to notice their attempts at engagement. As he got older, Patricia reports that Jacob appeared to become more interested in peers; however, peer interactions rarely ended well. Jacob had difficulty initiating interactions with others, often "bossing the other kids around." Jacob was intolerant with games that the other kids "made up" and imaginary play, frequently getting into arguments with peers and insisting that they were not playing "the right way." From an early age, Jacob had a fascination with trains, and Patricia notes that he would talk about trains incessantly. Trains have become a topic of irritation for Jacob's family because Patricia reports that he does not seem to recognize that others are not following or interested in the topic. Jacob will have one-sided conversations about trains and does not seem to understand that others have different interests from his. Jacob has not expanded his interests and seemingly resists all attempts to engage him in other topics.

At home, Jacob's mom reports that the family feels as though they are walking on eggshells all the time. Jacob is demanding and bossy, frequently throwing "fits" when things do not go the way he wants. His mom reports that Jacob will scream, cry, and throw objects at the slightest provocation. She also reports that Jacob's need for consistency and routine has caused significant turmoil within the family. Problematic situations can include things like moving the furniture to accommodate the Christmas tree; changing brands of food, laundry detergent, or personal products; or even the changes in the route taken to school. Patricia admits that she frequently gets frustrated with his sister's refusal to adhere to some of Jacob's specifications, which has caused animosity and discord within the family unit.

Recently, Jacob has been having difficulty in school, particularly with his peers. Jacob has begun expressing dissatisfaction with his peers' behavior during class as well as a lack of friends. Patricia reports that Jacob seems to be unhappy and is concerned that his "selfishness" has affected his ability to make and keep friends. Per teacher report, Jacob has difficulty with peers who do not adhere to the rules of the classroom. Jacob will tell on his peers, even his "friends," if they talk when they are not supposed to be talking or for any other slight infractions. His teacher refers to him as a "rule follower." Jacob's teacher reports that he is often alone during recess despite his awkward attempts to initiate interactions with others. Jacob's teacher reports that his attempts to engage with his peers are often disruptive and off-putting to others. When she approached the topic with Jacob, he did not seem to understand why his peers may be upset with him for telling on them when he was "just telling the truth." Jacob struggles with group work because he is inflexible with ideas and often tries to dictate how and what the group will do. Jacob's teacher reports spending inordinate amounts of time helping his groups resolve conflicts for which he is responsible. When the students are given the opportunity to choose their own groups, Jacob is frequently left out. Jacob blames the children for being "mean" and purposefully excluding him. He frequently yells at his peers, accusing them of "bullying" and demanding to be in their group and threatening to report them to the antibullying task force.

In addition to difficulties with peers in the school setting, Jacob's teacher reports that his grades are suffering. Jacob frequently argues with his teacher about the accuracy of tests, papers, and work materials. Jacob struggles to complete creative writing assignments, refusing to "make things up" and insisting on providing "real" and "right" information. For example, Jacob's teacher reported that when given the writing prompt: "If you could have a super power what would it be and why?" Jacob argued the plausibility of such a thing and refused to complete the assignment. Jacob also argued with peers about their assignments, telling them that it is not real and that it could not happen. Despite his difficulties in the academic realm, both his teacher and his mother report that Jacob's ability far exceeds his current level of functioning.

Jacob presented with his mom for the second session. Jacob greeted the counselor by stating that he did not know why he had to come and that he is not the one with the "problems." When asked why he thought that his mom brought him, he stated that he "didn't know." Jacob did not make eye contact and moved about the room picking up and touching objects. When asked to describe the "problems" that others have with him, he reported that the kids in his class are mean and stupid. Jacob reported that he wants to have friends but that there are not many good ones in his school. Jacob reported that they do not talk to him and that no one plays with him. During the session, Jacob was given the opportunity to play with various toys and games. Jacob took control of the play tasks, telling his mom and the counselor how to play by using statements such as "that's not right," "this is what you're supposed to do," and "stop it." When Jacob encountered something that he did not agree with or something that was not "right," he criticized the counselor by using statements such as "don't you know anything?" and "aren't you supposed to be smart?" When asked to speculate how others may feel when he uses such statements, Jacob responded that he did not know. When asked how he would feel, Jacob stated that it never happened, so he does not know. When asked to guess, Jacob became frustrated and irritated and told the counselor, "This is stupid. I'm not talking about this anymore."

■ DIAGNOSTIC IMPRESSIONS

Jacob demonstrates deficits in social communication and social interaction across multiple contexts including: deficits in social–emotional reciprocity by history and continuing in the present, demonstrated by abnormal, often intrusive and disruptive, social approach, failure of normal back-and-forth conversation, failure to respond to social interactions, and reduced sharing of interests and emotions; deficits in nonverbal communicative behaviors for social interaction—abnormalities in eye contact; and deficits in developing, maintaining, and understanding relationships demonstrated by difficulties with adjusting behaviors to suit various social contexts, difficulties with imaginative play, and difficulties making friends. Jacob also demonstrates restrictive, repetitive patterns of behavior, interests, and activities demonstrated by insistence on sameness and inflexible adherence to routine reflected in his "rule-following" and bossy behavior with peers and his history of strong preference for specific objects (cup) or brands. In addition, Jacob's intense interest in trains is a highly restricted, fixated interest that is abnormal in intensity and focus. Jacob's symptoms presented in the early developmental period and have created a clinically significant impairment in social and academic functioning in multiple settings.

■ DIAGNOSTIC CONCLUSION

Autism Spectrum Disorder (ASD) requiring support for deficits in both social communication and restricted repetitive behaviors, without accompanying intellectual impairment and without accompanying language impairment.

■ SUGGESTED THERAPEUTIC INTERVENTIONS

Family/Individual Therapy—Individual sessions with parents to educate the parent's about the symptoms, causes, and treatments of ASD. Assist the family in developing realistic expectations based on Jacob's abilities. Individual sessions with parents will also be used to teach behavior management skills to increase prosocial behaviors and decrease disruptive behaviors. Family sessions should be utilized, with all members present, to share and work through their feelings related to the impact that ASD has on the family.

Individual Therapy—Research demonstrates that the use of cognitive behavior therapy (CBT) for children with ASDs is effective in reducing the symptoms of anxiety and also has an impact on issues with social cognition (Kincade & McBride, 2009). Individual therapy with Jacob should focus on emotion identification and expression, perspective taking, and to develop prosocial coping skills.

School Collaboration—Therapist should assist the parents in collaborating with the school to develop a behavioral management system in the classroom to reinforce appropriate behavior and to improve school performance. In order to increase communication between the school and home, a communication system should be established (i.e., daily behavior reports). In addition, Jacob should participate in a school-based social group (e.g., a lunch bunch) to facilitate appropriate peer interaction.

Social/Peer Relationship Building—Involvement in a child-based social skills group program that focuses on peer relationships will assist Jacob in developing and maintaining appropriate friendships. The program should not occur without simultaneous parent behavior management training and ongoing collaboration with the program instructors.

■ FOR YOUR CONSIDERATION

1. What other information would you like to know in determining the best course of treatment for Jacob?
2. How do the family dynamics presented contribute to Jacob's difficulties?
3. What other courses of treatment may you suggest?

■ REFERENCE

Kincade, S. R., & McBride, D. L. (2009). CBT and autism spectrum disorders: A comprehensive literature review. Retrieved from http://files.eric.ed.gov/fulltext/ED506298.pdf

CASE TWENTY–EIGHT

Jason

■ HISTORY

Jason is a 23-year-old gay male who has recently graduated from college for sports management. While attending college, Jason found himself engaging in various sexual activities with a multitude of partners, claiming he was always safe, used protection, and got tested regularly for sexually transmitted diseases. Jason remarks that his sexual history was relatively normal until he met his now longtime boyfriend Mark. After having numerous sexual encounters with Mark, Jason started experiencing difficulty maintaining an erection during sexual acts with Mark, causing great strain on their relationship. Mark constantly remarks to Jason that he feels he "doesn't find him attractive anymore," whereas Jason continuously validates Mark's attractiveness to him.

Jason has come to therapy hoping for a solution to his sexual dilemma as a recommendation from his primary care physician (PCP). Jason explains that his PCP had found no biological reason behind his erectile dysfunction and that he should seek counseling to see if any mental health strategies could be implemented to alleviate his issue. Jason explains that this issue has lasted for the past 9 months of his relationship with Mark, roughly starting 6 months after the beginning of their relationship. While going over their relationship, Jason explains that until this issue appeared, he and Mark were extremely happy and carefree. Both had gotten an apartment together and found great jobs out of school, and Mark had a great relationship with Jason's parents.

Jason explains that in the last month, his work schedule has caused his and Mark's relationship to be further strained, causing Jason to drop interest in his fantasy football league that he and Mark both ran with a mutual friend group. Jason explains that since his shift in work a month ago, he has felt even more sad and hopeless with his relationship with Mark, expressing how much he loves him, but that he does not feel he can fix the rift he feels in their relationship. Jason also remarks that he never feels "fully focused" at work and that he is never able to concentrate fully on his work like he had been able to in the past. Because of these stressors, Jason explains that he "lies awake at night, thinking about all of the aspects of his life that are going wrong" and that he has found he loses more and more sleep each night. During a session with both Jason and Mark, Mark commented "how much less energy and passion Jason seems to have lately" and that he seems to "not be able to make up his mind" when given choices.

After much questioning, Jason and Mark finally reveal more personal details about Mark and his sexual relationship, explaining that his erectile dysfunction happens no matter what kind of sexual act he and Mark are performing. Mark explains that the issue has caused strain on his relationship with Jason but that he is even more concerned with Jason's mental health as of late than the lack of sexual intimacy. Jason explains how he does not feel "like the man Mark needs" in his life because he is unable to pleasure him physically, mentally, and emotionally.

Jason explains that Mark is a very strong-willed individual and can be very blunt with criticism. Beyond this, Jason remarks that Mark is "nearly perfect for me. We always seem to be on the same page, and we both have goals and desire to achieve them together in life. Whenever I feel down, Mark is always there to try to support me and help me. The only thing about Mark I would like to change is how blunt he can be with his words." Jason explains that Mark can try to be dominating whenever Jason is working on a project or when they are partaking in sexual activities. Jason explains that within the last month, Mark has also made very blunt statements about his changes in mood and behavior, causing Jason to feel less open to explain to Mark his feelings of hopelessness and sadness for fear of criticism from Mark.

■ DIAGNOSTIC IMPRESSIONS

When it comes to a relationship and sexual encounters, there is a level of nervousness that is normal, and individuals may report that there may be difficulty coping with the anxiety and anticipation in order to enjoy the experience. As is the case with many Erectile Dysfunction cases, something is blocking a person's ability to enjoy and partake in the sexual experience, be it trauma, self-confidence issues, or something undetermined. With this disorder, the occurrence of distress and issue happens nearly always with the individual, and this disorder can come paired with other issues.

Jason experiences great difficulty with his Erectile Dysfunction, and as such it starts to take a toll on the rest of his life. As this issue lasts longer and longer, his relationship with Mark falls apart to an ever increasing degree. Because of the stress associated with the Erectile Dysfunction, coupled with his work stress, he begins to develop symptoms of depression, further hurting his relationship and creating more concern for his mental well-being. Jason experiences feelings of sadness and hopelessness rather often with all of the stressors in his life. He also starts to lose interest in his favorite activities and feels a loss of energy and general sleep health. Finally, his depressive symptoms have caused him to have difficulty maintaining his concentration at work, further exacerbating his feelings of hopelessness.

■ DIAGNOSTIC CONCLUSIONS

Individuals with Erectile Dysfunction Disorder may find themselves with other comorbid conditions. For Erectile Dysfunction to be the true diagnosis, the individual must experience the issue more than 70% of the time during sexual interactions, for at least 6 months. This dysfunction must not be better explained by a mentally distressing event or from severe relationship distress. Also, for the dysfunction to be diagnosed, it must cause severe impairment in a client's life. Without these criteria being met, the dysfunction may stem from a lack of self-confidence, trauma and abuse, or can be better explained by substance abuse.

Major Depressive Disorder involves meeting the criterion of at least five of nine different symptoms that can manifest in a client's life, and these five symptoms must also be seen within a 2-week period for the diagnosis to be made. With Major Depressive Disorder, individuals must also not have any schizophrenic-related disorders that would better explain the symptoms or major depressive episode that the client may be experiencing.

Individuals with depression may lack the confidence to maintain an erection, while the lack of the ability to maintain an erection may cause more depressive feelings and ultimately be the true cause of the depressive episode.

Erectile Dysfunction Disorder
Major Depressive Disorder, Recurrent Episode, Moderate

■ SUGGESTED THERAPEUTIC INTERVENTIONS

Traditional counseling methods involving empathy and validation would be effective in pinpointing the direct cause of the erectile dysfunction. Jason most likely can pinpoint when the erectile dysfunction began, and with a strong rapport may be able to go into more detail around the mental processes that happen while performing sexual acts that cause the loss of his erection. Sex therapy may also be used to help address relationship issues that may be contributing to the dysfunction, noted heavily in the case study with Mark's blunt criticism.

Cognitive behavioral therapy may be utilized to help dispel negative thinking, behavioral, and systematic patterns to help reduce the symptoms of the depression. The fact that both partners also are trying to help salvage the relationship means that validating the clients through their depressive thoughts may allow them to see the supports that they have more clearly, creating stronger support networks for the client to navigate when depressive episodes strike, or even before, to help the client remain above the depression.

With this kind of delicate case in which the information is personal and relatively secretive, a strong rapport is necessary for therapy to be most effective. Individuals do not always share their sexual experiences (especially embarrassing or troublesome ones) lightly, which requires the counselor to have a strong rapport with his or her client. Owing to the coexistence of the depression in this case, the counselor will have to go below the depressive emotions and behaviors to find the true source of the client's erectile dysfunction, another layer of difficulty posed in the treatment of the client.

■ FOR YOUR CONSIDERATION

1. Could Jason's erectile dysfunction stem from a previous, albeit minor, major depressive episode that went undetected? If so, how could this change the diagnosis at hand, and how would treatment need to change, if at all, to address this difference?
2. How well do you think Mark will react to the idea that his harsh criticism could be the cause of Jason's worsening condition?
3. Could the idea of commitment be causation for Jason's erectile dysfunction given his freer nature throughout college?
4. Would this idea be worth pointing out to the client, or would this cause more difficulties in the already strained relationship?
5. Is this case more of a relationship dysfunction or an individual dilemma? Would therapy be more productive with both Jason and Mark present in each therapy session, or in this case would individual therapy with Jason be most beneficial?

Bashir

■ HISTORY

Bashir is a 19-year-old biracial (African American and Caucasian) male. He is currently unemployed and possesses a high school diploma. Bashir was adjudicated on charges of possession with intent to distribute, grand theft, destruction of property, and assault, after he had run away from home at the age of 17 years. He was caught by police after his parents reported Bashir as missing for several days. He was referred to treatment from a secure residential treatment facility to continue intensive outpatient treatment as he transitions from placement into a less-restrictive environment. This is Bashir's first foray into therapy.

Bashir does not know his biological parents because they never had custody. (Bashir was a premature baby and tested positive for drugs; he went immediately to foster care.) His first foster mother filed papers to adopt Bashir when he was a toddler (aged 2 years), but she was shot and killed by a boyfriend. Bashir was in the room when this happened. He was then placed with another foster family and their two older male children. He was eventually adopted by the couple. He reports that the household was stable, loving, but very strict. He shared that he never felt good enough for the family even though they were very supportive and kind to him. He noted that his adoptive family is Caucasian and he is biracial but looks more African

American. He said that strangers would ask his parents, "Where did he come from?" when he was a child, and he would feel embarrassed.

Bashir was on the honor roll in high school before he joined a gang to have a sense of belonging. In the background file that accompanied the referral, an interview with Bashir's adoptive mother reported that he went from being a good kid to one who was always high or drunk, disobeyed curfew and other rules, and stopped caring about doing well in school. She noted that Bashir would give himself tattoos and piercings in visible areas (like his arms). She also reported that she once walked in on Bashir in the bathroom and he had what she thought were cuts all over his chest and abdomen. When she asked about the marks, Bashir brushed off her concerns.

He earned his high school diploma in placement. This bothers Bashir because he views "placement school" as less-than given his pregang aspirations to attend college and become a teacher. In addition, prior to being charged, he had impregnated his girlfriend who gave birth while Bashir was in placement. The child, a son, is now 16 months old. Bashir has infrequent contact with his ex-girlfriend and has never met his son. He expresses regret that he will not be there for his son just like his biological parents were not there for him, and he wonders if that is for the best.

Per the rules around his release and his ex-girlfriend's request for child support, Bashir will have to find employment. His probation officer and staff at the residential treatment facility found him a job at a fast food restaurant. Bashir got into an argument with a manager and quit 4 days into employment.

■ DIAGNOSTIC IMPRESSIONS

Bashir presents as moderately depressed (exhibits feelings of unhappiness, frustration over even small matters, increased cravings for food and weight gain, irritability, etc.). An appointment was made with the psychiatrist so that Bashir may perhaps be placed on medication. However, when the appointment was over, Bashir threw away the script for Zoloft. When asked why he did so, he replied that he does not want to be on medication because that would make him weak.

He also does not see the difference between using drugs on the street and using drugs that are prescribed by a physician.

Bashir is proud of his tattoos and when asked "if they hurt," he noted that pain is the entire point. Bashir seems proud of his ability to withstand physical pain, and he derives positive feelings from the pain. When asked about other forms of self-injury, he said that he might have cut himself in the past but no longer does so. It should be noted, however, that Bashir has tattoos covering his arms, hands, neck, and ear. He also has piercings in his lip, ear, nose, and brow. He seems to endorse self-injury as a way to cope with intense emotional distress.

Bashir has unresolved attachment issues as evidenced by his developmental and preadoption history. Even though he was adopted into a loving family, he had a sense that he did not belong, and it seems to have been an overarching theme throughout his life. It seems that he always kept his adoptive family at arm's length so as to not be hurt by them. Further, he does not know his infant son and fears that he could be re-creating a destructive pattern for him.

■ DIAGNOSTIC CONCLUSIONS

Major Depressive Disorder, Moderate
Nonsuicidal self-injury
Lack of coping skills, problems with the legal system, and
difficulty with social supports

■ SUGGESTED THERAPEUTIC INTERVENTIONS

Psychopharmacology—Encourage Bashir to reconsider using medication to help his symptoms of depression.

Intensive Outpatient Therapy (2 to 3 days per week)—to comply with rules and expectations in the community consistently. Bashir will need to identify situations, thoughts, and feelings that trigger feelings of anger, frustration, or sadness, problem behaviors, and the targets of those actions. Assist Bashir in making connections

157

between his feelings and behavior. Use instruction, talk therapy, and/ or role-playing to help develop Bashir's emotional regulation. Assist Bashir in reconceptualizing anger as involving different components (e.g., cognitive, physiological, affective, and behavioral).

Family Therapy/Reunification Planning—to resolve past childhood/ family issues, leading to less anger and frustration, and greater self-esteem, security, and confidence. Bashir's behaviors have developed, in part, as a means of coping with feelings of abandonment and childhood trauma.

■ FOR YOUR CONSIDERATION

1. Would you consider extreme tattooing and piercing as a form of self-injury? Why or why not?
2. How do you respond when a client displays symptoms of something that may be well managed with medication and he or she refuses?
3. When they do speak, Bashir often argues with his child's mother about his lack of involvement in the child's life. (He is in placement, and has been since before the child's birth.) How can Bashir be a part of his child's life without being present?

Index

acne medication, 140
ACT values clarification, 42
ADHD. *See* Attention-Deficit/
    Hyperactivity Disorder (ADHD)
Alcoholics Anonymous, 10
alcohol use, 7
  history of, 8
  treatment for, 8
Alcohol Use Disorder, 9, 10, 81
American Counseling Association
    Competencies for Counseling
    with Transgender Clients, 36
American Society of Addiction Medicine
    Patient Placement Criteria, 10
anger issues, probation for, 55
antidepressant-induced sexual
    dysfunction, 29–30
Antisocial Personality Disorder, 120
anxiety, 2, 19, 20, 22, 23, 25, 55, 91–92,
    102, 105
  coping with, 151
  health, 21–22
  personal and social, 132
  primary care physician for, 105
  symptoms of, 1, 147
appetite loss, 9
apprehensive expectation, 91–92
arrestable behaviors, 119
ASD. *See* Autism Spectrum Disorder
    (ASD)
assault, 83
  treatment, 85

asthma, 40
attachment issues, 157
Attention-Deficit/ Hyperactivity
    Disorder (ADHD), 40, 66, 98, 114
  diagnoses of, 68
Autism, 40
Autism Spectrum Disorder (ASD), 4, 68,
    106, 147

behavior, 43
  management, 66, 147
  modification, 4, 114, 128
  problems, 66
behavioral therapy, 5
blackouts, 9
BM. *See* behavioral management (BM)
Borderline Personality Disorder (BPD),
    58
  symptoms of, 59
BPD. *See* Borderline Personality
    Disorder (BPD)
breathing
  exercise, 17
  techniques, 57

CBT. *See* cognitive behavioral therapy
    (CBT)
Celebrate Recovery, 10
chest pain, 106
childhood abuse, 9
childhood trauma, 102
Children's Services, 16

Child Sexual Abuse, 46–47
    diagnosis of, 47
chronic alcoholic, 7
citalopram, 27
cirrhosis, 8
cognitive behavioral strategies, 105–106
cognitive behavioral therapy (CBT), 10,
        21, 25, 73, 86, 128, 133, 152
    for children with ASDs, 147
    elements of, 11
    interventions, 113–114
    techniques, 42
    use of, 92
comorbidity, 124
compulsions, 132
Conduct Disorder, 110, 111, 113
conflicted relationships, 117–119
coping, 102–103
    with anxiety, 151
    mechanism, 91–92
    skills, 57, 74, 78
counseling process, 46

DBT. *See* dialectical behavior therapy
        (DBT)
decision-making skills, 78
delusion, 68, 73, 76–77
    of persecution, 69
Delusional Disorder, 72–73, 76–77
depression, 19, 20, 22, 23, 27, 68, 89,
        156–157
    coexistence of, 153
    individuals with, 152
    symptoms of, 34, 115
depressive cognitions, 29
dialectical behavior therapy (DBT), 44,
        59, 103
    self-management skills, 42
"different from the other kids," 143
distress tolerance skills, 60
drinking, 79
DSM-5 criteria for Excoriation (skin-
        picking) Disorder, 140–141
Dyspraxia, 40

eating disordered behaviors, 40
eating disorders, treatment of, 39
ED. *See* erectile dysfunction (ED)
emotional abuse, 99
emotional distress, 59
enuresis, 15–16
erectile dysfunction (ED), 28, 150–152
Erectile Dysfunction Disorder, 151–152
exposure therapy, 25
extraneous stimuli, 97

Family Acceptance Project, 36
family counseling, 17
family therapy, 36, 68–69, 74, 107, 147, 158
fatigue, 24
Female Sexual Arousal Disorder, 124
Female Sexual Distress Scale—Revised
        (FSDS-R), 125–126
female sexual dysfunction (FSD),
        124, 126
Female Sexual Interest/Arousal
        Disorder, 126, 127
    DSM-5 criteria for, 128
FSD. *See* female sexual dysfunction (FSD)

gastrointestinal problems, 41
GED. *See* general educational
        development (GED)
Gender Dysphoria in Adolescents, 35
gender role, 127
general educational development
        (GED), 11
generalized anxiety disorder, 25, 92
group therapy, 25

habit reversal training (HRT), 4
health anxiety, 21–22
heart palpitations, 106
heterosexual, 131
hopelessness, 151
HRT. *See* habit reversal training (HRT)
human needs, 13
hyperactivity, 97
hypertension, 27

illegal behavior, 117–119
impulsive aggressive outbursts, 112
impulsivity, 97
inattention, 97
individual therapy, 92, 147
ineffective modalities, 69
intense pain, 20
intensive outpatient therapy,
    157–158
Intermittent Explosive Disorder,
    111, 112–113
Internalized Homophobia, 132
intimacy, 28
irritability, 71

lesbian, gay, bisexual, transgender, and
    queer (LGBTQ) children, 36
LGBTQ children. *See* lesbian, gay,
    bisexual, transgender, and queer
    (LGBTQ) children

Major Depressive Disorder, 35, 68,
    110, 152
  diagnosis of, 111
  symptoms of, 111
Major Neurocognitive Disorder (NCD),
    80–81
maladaptive behavior patterns, 10
marijuana, 101
masculine clothing, 34
medication, 156–157
  management, 74
meditation, mindfulness, 128
mental distress, 60
mental health
  counseling for pain management, 20
  disorders, 40
  strategies, 149
  symptoms, 100
mental well-being, 151
MI. *See* motivational interviewing (MI)
mindfulness meditation, 128
motivational interviewing (MI), 10
motivation, lack of, 65

NA. *See* Narcotics Anonymous (NA)
Narcissistic Personality Disorder (NPD),
    73, 85–86, 120
Narcotics Anonymous (NA), 103
narrative therapy, 36
nausea, 9
NCD. *See* Major Neurocognitive
    Disorder (NCD)
NICHQ Vanderbilt Assessment
    Scale, 112
nonarrestable behaviors, 119
nonsuicidal self-injury (NSSI), 49
NPD. *See* Narcissistic Personality
    Disorder (NPD)
NSSI. *See* nonsuicidal
    self-injury (NSSI)

obesity, 27, 28
obsessions, 132
Obsessive Compulsive Disorder (OCD),
    4, 100
  diagnoses of, 68
  manifestation of, 132
  severity of, 5
  symptoms of, 4, 5, 22, 66, 113–114
  treatment of, 5
OCD. *See* Obsessive Compulsive
    Disorder (OCD)
ODD. *See* Oppositional Defiant Disorder
    (ODD)
Oppositional Defiant Disorder (ODD),
    66, 113
  diagnoses of, 68
  diagnosis, 114
  symptoms of, 112, 115
orthodontia, 39
outpatient therapy, 133

"pain all over," 19
pain management, mental health
    counseling for, 20
Panic Disorder, 107
paranoia, 69, 76–77
paranoid symptomatology, 75

paraphilic disorder, 136
    treatment success of, 86
PCP. *See* primary care physician (PCP)
peer/peering, 65, 135, 143, 145
    behavior, 144
    relationships, 140
person-centered therapy, 44
pervasive depressive symptoms, 68
pharmacotherapy, 68, 92, 98
physical abuse, 99
physical contact, 131
physical distress, 60
physical fitness, 89
physical intimacy, 124, 125
physical sex, 83
pigmentation, 139
pornography, 136
positive coping skills, 102–103
Posttraumatic Stress Disorder (PTSD), 9,
    11, 46, 48, 58, 100, 101, 126
    criteria for, 47
    diagnosis of, 46–47, 57, 58
    symptoms, 49–50
primary care physician (PCP), 149
problem-solving strategies, 78
prolonged illness, 1
prosocial coping skills, 147
prostitution, 8
psychoeducation, 22
psychopharmacology, 107, 133,
    137, 157
psychotherapy, 27
    treatment options, 127
PTSD. *See* Posttraumatic Stress Disorder
    (PTSD)
public drunkenness, 79–80
RAD. *See* Reactive Attachment Disorder
    (RAD)
Reactive Attachment Disorder (RAD),
    15–17
relationship issues, 58

relaxation
   skills, 50
   techniques, 57
reluctance, 109
repetitive behaviors, 132
restlessness, 9
restrictive eating behaviors, 41
reunification planning, 158

sadness, 9, 151
Schizoaffective Disorder, 66–67
Schizophrenia, 77
   diagnosis of, 68
school collaboration, 147
selective mutism, 44
selective serotonin reuptake inhibitors
    (SSRIs), 133
   antidepressants, 29, 30
self-calming skill development, 43
self-care, 43
self-esteem, 125
self-harming behavior, 46, 48–49, 58
self-injury, 157
self-management, 44
sensate focus techniques, 128
sense of belonging, 156
separation anxiety, 66
Severe Alcohol-induced Major
    Neurocognitive Disorder, 81
Severe Sexual Sadism Scale (SSSS), 86
sex, 125
sexual abuse, 14, 15, 45–49, 55–57, 59
   disclosure of, 57
   experiences, 59
sexual activities, 149, 150
sexual arousal, 83, 85
sexual assault, 7–9
sexual contact, 131
sexual dysfunction, 28, 29
   female, 124
   prevalence of, 124

sexual interactions, 151
sexually transmitted diseases, 149
Sexual Orientation Obsession, 132
sexual physical contact, 125
sexual problems, 123
sexual relationships, 135–136
Sexual Sadism, 86
  criteria for, 85
  prevalence of, 86
sexual trauma, 57
social communication, deficits in, 146
social interaction, deficits in, 146
social/peer relationship building,
  98, 147
Somatic Symptom Disorder, 20, 22
SSRIs. *See* selective serotonin reuptake
  inhibitors (SSRIs)
SSSS. *See* Severe Sexual Sadism Scale
  (SSSS)
stomach flu, 1
  symptoms, 3
stress, 51, 151
  management, 50
substance abuse, 57
  impulsive behaviors of, 58
  issues, 57
Substance/Medication-induced Sexual
  Dysfunction, 28–30

substance use, 7, 58
  probation for, 55
Substance Use Disorders,
  126–127

temper outburst, 109
testosterone hormone therapy, 33
TF-CBT. *See* trauma-focused cognitive
  behavior therapy (TF-CBT)
Tic Disorder, 4
traditional counseling methods, 152
traditional empathic counseling,
  120–121
transgender children, 33–36
trauma-focused cognitive behavior
  therapy (TF-CBT), 49–52

upset, 13

valsartan, 27
Ventolin inhaler, 40
violent sexual act, 85
visualization, 50
vomiting, 1–3
voyeurism, 135, 136
voyeuristic disorder, 136

weight loss, symptoms, 2

Made in the USA
Las Vegas, NV
05 February 2022